# MENTAL HEALTH THROUGH NUTRITION

JUDGE TOM R. BLAINE

# Mental Health Through Nutrition

*Introduction by A. HOFFER, M.D., Ph.D.*

*THE CITADEL PRESS*
*Secaucus, New Jersey*

TO

*JOHN W. TINTERA, M.D.*

# CONTENTS

INTRODUCTION / 9

*Chapter One*
THE NEED FOR BETTER NUTRITIONAL EDUCATION / 17

*Chapter Two*
HOPE FOR THE MENTALLY ILL / 27

*Chapter Three*
HYPOGLYCEMIA—THE IGNORED DISEASE / 35

*Chapter Four*
VITAMINS BRING MENTAL HEALTH / 49

*Chapter Five*
SCHIZOPHRENIA, A PHYSICAL DISEASE THAT AFFECTS
THE MIND / 71

*Chapter Six*
SCHIZOPHRENIA RESPONDS FAVORABLY TO VITAMIN
THERAPY / 85

*Chapter Seven*
"YOU WILL NEVER KNOW THE HELL I ENDURED" / 97

*Chapter Eight*
HEALTH BONUSES GALORE / 125

*Chapter Nine*
PHYSICAL AND MENTAL HEALTH ASSURED / 141

*Appendix A*
THE FAT-SOLUBLE VITAMINS
THE WATER-SOLUBLE VITAMINS
TABLE OF VITAMINS IN FOODS / 151

*Appendix B*
DIETARY LEVELS OF HOUSEHOLDS IN THE UNITED
STATES, SPRING, 1965 / 177

*Appendix C*
TREATMENT OF SCHIZOPHRENIA / 187

*Appendix D*
GERIATRIC NUTRITION / 197

# INTRODUCTION

Recently, Professor Linus Pauling (*Science*, April, 1968, vol. 160, pp. 265-271) introduced a concept, orthomolecular psychiatry, which he defined as the treatment of mental disease by the provision of the optimum molecular environment for the mind, especially the optimum concentrations of substances normally present in the body. In the course of evolution, man's body lost the ability to make many important molecules, such as ascorbic acid, essential amino acids, and essential fatty acids, as they became available in his food. During evolution, endogenous synthesis gave way to a dependency upon external dietary sources. Until about 10,000 years ago, this did not create any major difficulty, because man's palate and the limited availability of foods rich in easily absorbed carbohydrates and sugars kept a proper balance between the evolutionary changes and food consumption. One might say that man either starved or ate well but that malnutrition was rare. Until a century ago this was still generally true of the Eskimo.

About 10,000 years ago, man discovered how to grow cereal crops, which soon provided an abundant supply of low-cost, easily available foods. As a result, there was an enormous increase in the population of the earth and the development of our urban societies became possible. It is inconceivable that cities could have arisen without the development of cereal agriculture as we know it today. However, man, whose body had adapted over several million years to a high-protein, high-fat diet (fresh meat, carrion, bugs, berries), now had to deal with an ever-increasing amount of carbohydrates, which in some diets today reaches 40 per cent of the total caloric intake. Man's palate still acted as a rough guide, since protein and fatty foods are generally more palatable than the starchy foods, such as potatoes, breads, corn, and rice, etc. However, in our Western culture another development began about twenty years ago which has removed even palatability as a guide. The food industries have discovered how to make even paper palatable. Skillful use of condiments and sugar removed man's last natural guide. As a result, in the United States, in England, and in Canada there has been an enormous increase in the consumption of high-calorie, low-vitamin and mineral foods, such as sugar, etc. There is thus a wide discrepancy between what the body requires and what our natural desires lead us to consume. Since man can no longer depend upon palatability as a guide, he must turn to his intelligence. He must intelligently select food which will keep his body and mind healthy. Unfortunately, this kind of nutrition is not taught in our schools, nor is it taught in our medical schools. It will be the function of orthomolecular physicians to practice this art.

Judge Tom R. Blaine's book *Mental Health Through Nutrition* might also be called *Orthomolecular Psychiatry for the Layman*. It is a remarkably clear and accurate exposition of the nutritional needs of man and must be followed rigorously if one is to achieve the optimum health which one's inheritance has programmed.

Judge Blaine makes the following charges:

1. That doctors who know anything about nutrition have not learned it from medical college.

2. That nutrition is ignored by most physicians.

3. That if the few simple rules of nutrition recommended are followed, there will be a major decrease in mental illness.

He has emphasized two main conditions which respond to better nutrition or to the use of megavitamin therapy. These are relative hypoglycemia, better called hyperinsulinism, and schizophrenia. These nutritional concepts, widely known and carefully described in the medical literature, are resisted stoutly by believers in the prevailing philosophy that all mental illnesses arise from problems in one's life, usually from bad fathering and/or bad mothering.

My associate Dr. Osmond and I can both testify to the truth of Judge Blaine's assertions. Although we have had powerful and enthusiastic support for our megavitamin $B_3$ work by men like Sir Julian Huxley, Dr. N. Lewis, and Professor H. Kluver, and more recently by Professor Linus Pauling, these brilliant, brave men stand alone among a vast majority of psychoanalytically-oriented teachers of psychiatry in our universities, whose main posture is that it is inconceivable that nutrition and vitamins can do what we found they *did* do.

Recently, an eminent professor of psychiatry lamented that not a single discovery in the field of psychiatry had been made by university departments of psychiatry nor were they teaching their students about the discoveries which had been made elsewhere.

My main interest in nutrition and vitamins did not come from my medical education but from my Ph.D. research on vitamins and cereal grains. During my medical education, we were given very little information about nutrition, except about bland and roughage diets. However, even with my basic appreciation of diets, it was not until three years ago that my good friend Dr. Robert Meiers of Twin Pines Hospital in Belmont, California, introduced me to the concept of hyperinsulinism. He was very enthusiastic about the results of diet treatment for it and infected me with his enthusiasm. A few days after returning to my office, a young woman came to consult me. She stated that she was sexually frigid and requested psychotherapy for the condition. This kind of problem is the psychoanalyst's dream, since it can lead to literally years of sexual interpretations. She seemed the most unlikely of all patients to have hyperinsulinism, but thinking that this might be a fine way to test Bob Meiers' hypothesis, I ordered a six-hour glucose tolerance test and also a malvaria urine test. To my great surprise, her blood sugar at four hours dropped to around 50 mg. and she also tested positive for malvaria. During her second interview, I introduced her to the diet concepts and started her on nicotinic acid, one gram taken three times a day, and ascorbic acid, one gram taken three times a day. She was given no psychotherapy of any dynamic sort. A month later she reported that frigidity was no longer a problem. When I asked her how she felt compared to a month before, she reported that she could not make such a comparison for she had been deeply depressed and tense all her life without knowing it, and only in the past two weeks had she discovered what it was like to be relaxed and at ease. A few months later, doubting that the diet could be quite so important and since it was Christmas, she began to eat excessive quantities of pastry and cakes. Within a few days she was deeply depressed, whereupon she quickly went back on her diet.

Since then I have examined hundreds of patients and have found, as have many others, that every alcoholic tested had hypoglycemia. There was really no point in testing them any further, since there were no exceptions. In addition, 75 per cent of the neurotics and schizophrenics who came to see me also had the same condition. Within the past two years it has become clearly evident in my own practice that 75 per cent of all the patients referred to me can be cured by a combination of proper diet and an adequate use of vitamin therapy, with tranquilizers and antidepressants as adjuncts.

It has also been gratifying to discover how quickly general practitioners who have referred their cases to me have learned to follow the same principles, and although this may not be good for my income, it is most gratifying to me as a research scientist.

*Mental Health Through Nutrition* is one of the few books written which relates mental health to nutrition and it may well remain a classic primer for everyone. Every doctor, nurse, dietitian, and every person directly involved in the care and treatment of the mentally ill must read this book. Every family which has a sick member in an institution, private or public, must read this book and see to it that the nutritional principles laid down by the author are followed by the institution.

Judge Blaine's book suggests that if every person from childhood on were given the proper nutrition and vitamin intake there might be a vast decrease in the incidence of all forms of mental illness. In fact, this is my belief too, and I have suggested elsewhere that if in our society we were to add larger quantities of vitamins to our food—for example, one gram of nicotinamide to the diet each day—then there is every possibility that within a matter of a decade or two there would be a major decrease in the incidence of alcoholism, schizophrenia, and perhaps other forms of mental illness. At least this is an experiment which should be tried, although the idea will be viewed as so far out that I doubt that it will be possible in my lifetime to have the experiment run.

ABRAM HOFFER, M.D., PH.D.

# MENTAL HEALTH THROUGH NUTRITION

# 1

# The need for better
# nutritional education

The curricula of most medical schools ignore the modern doctor's need for nutritional knowledge. In an editorial in the *Journal of the American Medical Association* (March 16, 1963), it was said:

"In general, medical education and medical practice have not kept abreast of the tremendous advances in nutritional knowledge. A recent survey by the Council on Foods and Nutrition on nutrition teaching in medical schools indicated that there is inadequate recognition, support and attention given to this subject in medical schools. . . . Undergraduate teaching of nutrition often is centered around nutritional deficiency diseases. This is too limited a focus for present-day problems. It is necessary to think more in terms of disturbances of the metabolic and biochemical reactions of the body."

In 1964, Helen Hair, a nutritionist at Jefferson Medical College in Philadelphia, spoke at the 13th Annual Pennsylvania Health Conference. She discussed the eating habits of medical students, and concluded they were as bad as the eating habits of older people. She said that 83 senior medical students at Jefferson tended to skip breakfast, ate food high in calories but nothing else, and believed they were getting adequate nutritional values.

She continued, "The medical students . . . seem to be more concerned with the caloric intake rather than whether they are obtaining adequate nutrition. Their attitude seems to be that they have been healthy and feel all right; therefore they must be getting good nutrition."

Dr. Willard A. Krehl, president of the American Society for Clinical Nutrition, recently said, "It is unfortunate that we have in our medical schools few, if any, professors of clinical nutrition." Dr. Krehl commented on the fact that many physicians are concerned that the teaching of nutrition is becoming weak in medical schools.

Most of the nation's leading nutritionists agree that there is a serious deficiency in the education of physicians in the area of nutrition.

Dr. Donald M. Watkin wrote in the April, 1965, issue of the *American Journal of Public Health* that despite nutrition's impact on medicine, it does not have a place in the curricula of more than a handful of medical schools. Other physicians have pointed out that formal nutritional courses are hard to find in medical schools.

Dr. Carl Lamb, of Philadelphia, told *Health Bulletin* in 1965 that he never asked medical students any questions on nutrition in a test or on a board examination. Dr. Lamb, whose specialty is obstetrics and gynecology, said that students were given nutritional manuals and expected to do research on their own. "Other than that," he said, "nutrition was never stressed."

Ogden C. Johnson, Ph.D., of the American Medical Association's Department of Food and Nutrition, said in the December, 1965, issue of *Nutrition Reviews*,

"Major medical and educational organizations have held meetings deploring the state of nutritional education in medical schools."

In setting up the curricula for medical schools, it is evident that physicians have overlooked the one point that Louis Pasteur so often emphasized: that it is far more important to prevent a disease than it is to treat it. It is obvious that most of the dreaded diseases that have been almost abolished from civilized races—such as plague, typhoid, cholera, malaria—have been controlled by preventative means and not by cure.

For years, nutritionists have known that sugar in moderation is a harmless enough food for most persons. They have also known that nearly all the infamous criminals of whose eating habits any records are available ate excessive amounts of sugar. When it was suggested to psychiatrists that sugar might be poisonous to some users, and that there was a possibility that sugar had something to do with the behavior of criminals, they ridiculed the suggestions. For years, anyone who intimated that faulty nutrition played any part in the mental processes of criminals and others who acted irrationally, was labeled a "food faddist," and the suggestion was dismissed as frivolous.

Dr. Marvin Ziporyn, the Chicago psychiatrist who visited Richard Speck almost twice a week before Speck's trial, recounted in his book *Born to Raise Hell* that Speck had a host of mental kinks, and that he munched on Baby Ruth candy bars. Dr. Ziporyn, a confessed disciple of Freud, found that this killer of eight student nurses was unable to control himself as a result of his emotional and medical past. In his book, Ziporyn advocated "rehabilitation over retribution" for Speck.

Dr. Francis Pottenger, Jr., a famous California child specialist, was interviewed a few years back by the *Daily News and Leader* (Springfield, Ill.) on the causes of juvenile delinquency. "If I were to name the chief cause of juvenile delinquency and of the growing crime rate, I would say it was malnutrition," said Dr. Pottenger.

Every authentic account of the life of Adolf Hitler indicates that he was a "sugar drunkard."

A staff writer on the Los Angeles *Herald Examiner* (August 12, 1962), in discussing the cases of the last four women executed for murder in California, discussed the eating habits of each woman, and concluded that the four were slaves to sugar.

The *London Mirror* gave an account of a paper read by Dr. Richard Mackarness on August 21, 1964, before the International Congress of Social Psychiatry in London. He told of a youthful delinquent whose diet consisted mostly of ice cream, cakes, chocolates, and other goodies. Dr. Mackarness reported that a week after all sugar products had been taken away from this boy, "he became as good as gold." To test his "cure," Dr. Mackarness permitted the boy to eat his sugared foods again, and within two days his conduct was as bad as before. When the sweets were once more removed, the youth again became an exemplary young man.

John Crosby, writing in the New York *Herald Tribune* on May 21, 1962, on the causes of juvenile delinquency and the solutions proposed, said, "The experts in juvenile delinquency are getting to be voodoo priests talking their own mumbo jumbo that doesn't seem to mean anything or apply to anything."

Some medical fallacies have either caused or contributed to the poor physical and mental health of Americans. We shall discuss a few of these fallacies.

*Fallacy No. 1. That the average American diet contains all the vitamins and minerals necessary for good health.* (Read Appendix B.)

The expression "average American diet" is merely a figment of the imagination. It is ridiculous to assume that any political authority or any medical specialist can set up a mathematical formula of food values that will apply to all. When we ignore the relationships between the condition of the various soils in which our foods are grown, the losses in nutritional value due to marketing, processing, storing, cooking, menu balancing, and, most important of all, the problems of food absorption by human bodies, either healthy or diseased, we see how foolish is the generally accepted view of physicians that we get a balanced food intake, containing all the vitamins and minerals necessary for health, in an "average American diet."

Dr. Frederick Kilander, of New York, after 28 years of study on the subject, declared that two out of three Americans cannot select a well-balanced meal in a cafeteria, even when cost is not involved.

Dr. Herbert Ratner, of the Stritch School of Medicine, Loyola University, recently declared that the United States is one of the worst countries in the world in which to have a nonserious illness. Dr. Ratner continued: "We are the wealthiest country in the world—yet one of the unhealthiest countries in the world. . . . Our gastrointestinal system operates like a sputtering gas engine. We can't sleep; we can't get going when we are awake. We have neuroses. . . . Neither our hearts nor our heads last as long as they should."

*Fallacy No. 2. That senility is synonymous with old age.* (See Chapter 8.)

This is both a medical and a legal fallacy. Webster's New International Dictionary says that senility is "old age or its physical and mental infirmities." Dorland's Illustrated Medical Dictionary (24th ed.) defines senility as "old age." Stedman's Medical Dictionary also states that senility is "old age." Bouvier's Law Dictionary refers to senility as "the state of being old." Ballentine's Law Dictionary calls senility "the mental condition of an old person."

In the recent court case of Parker vs. Parker, (Ark.) 331 S.W. (2) 694, senility is said to be "old age." The Alabama appellate court, in the case of Equitable Life Assurance Society vs. Garrett, 160 S. 776, after reviewing the medical evidence submitted, observed that senility is a disease resulting from old age.

An advanced state of senility is called "senile dementia" and is declared to be a form of insanity in both the medical textbooks and the reported appellate cases. Many writers have attempted to soften the term "senile dementia" by referring to it as "venerable insanity," apparently on the assumption that some of us might resent being called insane simply because we are old.

History does not agree with the theory of inevitable mental deterioration; many prominent men and women, down through the ages, have retained their mental faculties to advanced years.

As we shall later see, senility cannot at the present time be cured; however, it *can be prevented* from marring old age by the observation of proper living habits, which include, among other things, good nutrition.

*Fallacy No. 3. That hypoglycemia, or low blood sugar, sufferers should have sugar.*

After the publication of *Goodbye Allergies* (a study of low blood sugar) in 1965, the author received hundreds of letters from hypoglycemia patients all over the nation, stating that physicians had recommended the addition of sugar to their diets. That any medical doctor could be so poorly informed does not seem likely. But listen to this: Scores wrote that their physicians did not believe there was such a condition as low blood sugar; that hypoglycemia was only a fad or the product of the imagination, and to forget all about it!

For a doctor to prescribe sugar for hypoglycemia is to display the same degree of medical knowledge as to advise an emphysemia patient to smoke more cigarettes or an alcoholic to drink more liquor.

(Fallacy Number Three is further discussed in Chapter 3.)

With the knowledge of nutrition now available, there is no reason for us to have the fear of old age that people had twenty or thirty years ago. However, as Agnes Faye Morgan, of the University of California, noted in the June, 1962, issue of *The Gerontologist*, "It is, of course, never too late to mend one's nutritional ways, but the full protection which may be expected from wise food choices can be obtained only when those habits are adopted early in life."

It may safely be said that the changes, physical and mental, that we observe in the aged are caused mostly by typical American food habits. We get too many calories from the wrong foods.

No one can or hopes to avoid old age, but we can avoid being "old." We should never forget that everything does not have to go downhill with age.

Dr. Nathan W. Schock, head of the Gerontology Branch of the National Heart Institute, recently said: "Old people show more variety in their ability and physical powers than any other age group. We've found that the ability to do a job—except for one that requires unusual strength or dexterity—rarely depends on age alone. The mental process does not necessarily dim with age. Those who think more and work more retain their alertness and working ability the longest. When we see people who slow down with their years, they are not showing the effect of time itself, they are suffering from the cumulative effects of a lifetime of traumas that literally have wiped out a part of the individual. We hope to find a way to avoid such tragedy."

In addition to proper nutrition and adequate physical exercise, if one is to live to a ripe age and retain his mental faculties, he must get adequate sleep. According to *Rutgers Pharmacy Extension News* (June, 1965), a team of medical workers at Colgate University found that mental workers require more sleep than laborers, and that getting enough sleep usually means eight hours a day. The same publication carries a report of the result of a study made by University of Chicago investigators, who found that morale is a key to health and that idleness will cause one to deteriorate both mentally and physically.

We have observed from press statements and medical articles that we may expect a different type of physician to enter the psychiatric field from those who have heretofore become psychiatrists.

According to a report made to the American Psychiatric Association in Detroit by Dr. Daniel De Sole, an Albany, N.Y., psychiatrist, and Samuel Aaronson, psychiatrists commit suicide at a rate of 70 per 100,000, or four times the rate of the general white population.

A check of the obituaries of 287 young psychiatrists as listed in the *Journal of the American Medical Association* showed that 84 of the deaths, or nearly 30 per cent, were suicides.

Dr. Walter Freeman, Chief of Neurology at Santa Clara County Hospital in San Jose, California, expressed the opinion that some psychiatrists cannot bear "the intense emotional experience of undergoing psychoanalytic training." Stated another way, those doctors who took their own lives could not endure the psychoanalytic experience necessary to becoming a psychiatrist, with its insistence upon a thorough insight into one's own personality.

If medical students and physicians cannot bear undergoing personal psychoanalysis, how are mentally disturbed laymen expected to endure it?

# 2
# Hope for
# the mentally ill

We should bow our heads in shame for the treatment mankind has given the mentally ill.

In England in the 1700's, scant attention was given to the poor and unfortunate. In the early part of that century, by paying twopence, an outsider was permitted to enter an asylum and make sport of the lunatics! Crowds delighted in seeing these forlorn creatures suffer their taunts and jeers.

In the early days of our own country it was believed that the only way to cure an insane person was to bleed, beat, blister, and torture him until the "evil spirit that possessed him" went away. Within the lifetime of some still living, it was held that the proper treatment for one "out of his mind" was to scare him into his senses.

Then, for generations, the insane asylums became vast warehouses where helpless human beings were herded together, hidden and forgotten. Until the past few years, the attitude of many hospital personnel toward a mental patient was that of a callous jailer toward his prisoner. The patient was not considered a sick person, but one who had to be disciplined with straitjackets, handcuffs, straps, chains, and clubs. His court papers said he had been committed, but actually he had been sentenced to imprisonment until death. It has been less than fifteen years since we last read newspaper stories of mental patients being chained to walls, radiators, or whatever was available.

The tragedy of the situation in the years past was made worse because of a conspiracy of silence among attendants as to what went on behind the walls of our mental institutions. Threats of injuries to an attendant by other attendants if he told of witnessing inhuman acts of brutality were usually sufficient to prevent exposures. The author presided as trial judge in a criminal case several years ago, where the evidence showed that a husky male attendant in a state hospital stomped a helpless old man patient to death to show a new attendant how to "control" the patients in a particular ward.

Doctors estimate that about one third of our mental hospitals are fairly well run. Even now, in our better-run institutions, many of the older patients appear to be more vegetables than people.

The late President Kennedy informed Congress prior to the appointment of the Joint Commission on Mental Illness and Health in 1961 that at some time or other mental illness will afflict one out of every three American families.

Conditions in our hospitals for the mentally ill have definitely improved during the last few years. The use of psychiatric drugs, particularly tranquilizers, has in most instances replaced the jailhouse treatment of patients. More effort is being made to get patients out of the hospitals and back in the home or, if that is not possible, in nursing homes or other qualified places. No longer does a committed patient enter a mental hospital with no hope of ever leaving it.

The release of a patient from a mental hospital does not mean that he or she has recovered. With the over-crowded conditions prevailing in most state hospitals, patients are sent home when only slight improvement has occurred.

Frequently, a mentally disturbed person finds that he is mistreated and actually abused at home. All too often, relatives take the view that one released from a mental institution could act differently if he tried, and that some of his irrational ways result from pure cussedness. Instead of trying to help him regain his mental health, relatives assume that discipline is what the strangely acting one needs.

Court officials are familiar with the marks on the bodies of many of those who are brought into court for sanity hearings. It seems too horrible to be true that these unfortunate people should be beaten, kicked, or otherwise injured by relatives who frequently are more interested in getting them back in state hospitals than in having them in their homes.

The majority of those who are sent home from mental hospitals are not physically abused by relatives. Unfortunately, however, most relatives have unrealistic and distorted opinions as to the causes of mental illness and what should be done to help toward recovery. Some of the beliefs of those who live with the mentally ill are little more advanced than were the opinions of the American colonists as to the cause of abnormal mental reactions.

One who has a physical ailment usually gets the sympathy and help of those who are close to him. Superstition, ignorance, and false beliefs regarding mental illness can destroy the sympathy of a husband, wife, parent, brother, or sister toward a mentally unfortunate relative.

Another tragedy of mental illness has been the cost, in usually futile efforts, of having a patient who was permitted to go home from a hospital treated privately. With the medical fees frequently running from twenty to fifty dollars for each treatment, loving relatives have spent all their savings, gone heavily in debt, and then had to have the loved one recommitted to the mental institution.

The principal reason our mental hospitals have done so little to restore mental health to the unfortunate people committed to such hospitals is that many of the physicians and psychologists connected with these institutions are now, or were in the past, followers of Sigmund Freud.

Dr. Edward R. Pinckney, well-known California physician and author, in his book *The Fallacy of Freud and Psychoanalysis* makes these observations:

"To me, psychoanalysis is a hoax—the biggest hoax ever played on humanity. By showing who analysts are, how they work, what they believe, and what they have done, I hope to show Freud as a fraud. . . . Probably the biggest factor contributing to the psychoanalytic hoax is that analysts strive so desperately to label their exploitation as a science without fulfilling any of the postulates set down and accepted by scientists the world over which would qualify it as being truly scientific. . . .

"The Freudian psychoanalyst not only ignores all of

today's accepted medical science, but even refuses to apply to his patients the same science he will gratefully accept for himself and his own family when he suffers from illness. I do not know of a single case where a psychoanalyst, even one with a medical degree, performed a comprehensive physical examination before commencing analytic treatment. Furthermore, a true Freudian psychoanalyst cannot allow his patient to take any medicine for whatever condition is under consideration. . . .

"Biological psychiatry is rapidly achieving scientific proof that specifically contradicts the Freudian concepts of all mental illness being the results of infantile sexual trauma. . . . Facts serve to point out that much of the sexual perversions of man are created by psychoanalysts. . . . Homosexuality has become so overt, due to analytical thinking and writings which have wholly accepted Freud's belief that everyone has homosexual tendencies, that what was once an attitude to be ashamed of, is now influencing our lives."

Dr. Pinckney then shows how the Freudian preoccupation with sex was demoralizing Americans. "Only one woman out of several hundred I have talked with regarding psychoanalysis and divorces told me her analyst insisted on her staying married." This woman then explained to Dr. Pinckney that her analyst only wanted her to stay with her husband until the husband had paid for the completion of the analysis!

"Freud's basic concepts tend to destroy any man-woman relationship," Dr. Pinckney continues. "The end result of a marriage plunged into an analytical morass must be divorce. . . . Marriage counselors who have had a high rate of success in rejoining 'broken homes' have told me that in their practical, actual experience, psychoanalysis does more to defeat marriage than the original, seemingly intolerable situation which initiated the conjugal dissolution.

"Freudian doctrine does serve as one more piece of evidence in the overall thesis that psychoanalysis serves only to lower standards of morality, or to eliminate the concept of conscience altogether. Can there be any justification—scientific, theological, or even sociological—for the promotion of promiscuity? Coming back to the prostitute [the ideal woman, according to Freud], is this way of life the ultimate goal of mankind?"•

When we think of our mental hospitals being staffed with men and women who share the weird views of Freud, is it any wonder that so little has been done for those in these hospitals?

One of the new tools used in our hospitals for the insane is "friendliness" toward patients. The medical world refers to this more humanitarian attitude with helpless persons as T.L.C.—tender, loving care. College students have been recruited all over America as volunteers to assist the attendants, nurses, therapists, and physicians. The heads of some of our better-run mental hospitals readily admit that the work of these volunteer college students has helped make the difference between success

• All of the quotations from *The Fallacy of Freud and Psychoanalysis* are with the permission of the author, Dr. Edward R. Pinckney, who is the owner of the copyright (1966). This book is available at cost by sending $3.00 to American Schizophrenia Foundation, 305 S. State Street, Ann Arbor, Michigan, 48108. Proceeds are donated to the Foundation.

and failure. These "college kids" are far more successful than the regular employees of the hospitals in getting patients interested in some kind of work or play therapy that will bring them back to a world of reality from their flight into a world of fantasy.

This much is certain: The mental hospitals of the future will not be the prisons and torture houses of yesterday. Custodial care, even with the help of tranquilizers and other psychiatric drugs, will give way to new treatment techniques which will recognize the mentally ill as persons sick in body and mind, but who can be cured.

The hospitals of tomorrow will not have on their staffs psychoanalysts who appear to take a fiendish delight in separating couples and in destroying marriages.

Instead of having large wards where a hundred mental patients can be stored away as if they were so many crates or bottles, big mental hospitals hundreds of miles away will be replaced by smaller, homelike hospitals in the patient's own community.

Canada's province of Saskatchewan has two mental hospitals. Dr. Fred Grunberg, superintendent of the hospital at Weyburn, permits patients to come and go as they please, shopping or visiting downtown, so long as they remain within the hours set by the ward staff. There are fewer escapes than when the wards were locked. The Saskatchewan government has equipped these hospitals so that the furnishings in the wards compare favorably with those of the most modern hotels in any modern city. Untrained, incompetent, and coldhearted attendants and nurses have been replaced by persons who are as competent and anxious to help patients recover as those in any other hospital.

In the Saskatchewan mental hospitals when a patient does not behave properly, a threat that he will be sent out of the hospital is usually all that is necessary to get him back in line.

To sum it up, mental hospitals will be built, staffed, and run to help, not to hurt, patients. Effective and humane treatment of these sick people will send them back home as soon as they are ready, without any stigma being attached to them, and jobs and homes will rehabilitate them in the shortest possible time.

When will all this happen? It will come when the people demand good mental hospitals with the same standards of medical care and nursing provided in hospitals for the physically ill. As we shall later see, this may be in a much shorter time than most of us have thought possible.

# 3
# Hypoglycemia—the ignored disease

Hypoglycemia is a low blood sugar condition, the opposite of hyperglycemia, a condition in which there is excess sugar in the bloodstream.

"Hyperinsulinism" is a medical term used to describe a condition caused by an excessive secretion of insulin by those parts of the pancreas called the islands of Langerhans. Unfortunately, many members of the medical profession refuse to accept the term hyperinsulinism, preferring to call the condition "relative hypoglycemia." It was interesting to note in some recent medical articles that the terms "functional hyperinsulinism" and "relative hypoglycemia" were used interchangeably.

Hypoglycemia is the opposite of diabetes (high blood sugar resulting from an insufficient secretion of the hormone insulin). Hypoglycemia, which is the result of too much insulin, has been called the hunger disease, the starvation disease, and the fatigue disease. An abnormal craving for sugar is a common characteristic of low blood sugar. Chronic fatigue is the usual complaint.

Doctors estimate there may be three to six times as many sufferers from low blood sugar as there are known diabetics, yet low blood sugar continues to be largely ignored by the men and women of medical science.

When we consider the seriousness of low blood sugar, it is difficult to understand why hypoglycemics have, for the most part, been tossed into the medical wastebaskets. Many honest physicians frankly tell their patients, when asked about low blood sugar, that they don't know how to diagnose and treat hypoglycemia. Other doctors will say that hypoglycemia is a fad that should be forgotten.

The layman does not understand why some physicians are prejudiced against hypoglycemia. The fact that it was not taught in medical schools is not sufficient reason for such a serious disturbance to be ignored. If doctors would only think of hypoglycemia as they do other bodily ailments, they might be able to diagnose it more readily and learn how to treat it effectively.

Although many excellent articles have appeared in recent years in the medical journals explaining why hypoglycemia sufferers cannot eat quickly absorbed carbohydrate foods, many doctors still prescribe sugar for hypoglycemia. This is the worst thing they could do, since sugar primes the pancreas to secrete more insulin and makes the hypoglycemia worse. The well-informed physician will treat hypoglycemia with a low carbohydrate and high protein diet. He knows that unless the patients are willing to change their eating habits—get off sugar and other quickly absorbed carbohydrates—they will continue to complain of fatigue, anxiety, nervousness, headaches, and to have mental confusion—sometimes with crying spells—and all kinds of allergic disorders.

The above are by no means all of the complaints of hypoglycemics. Doctors report that low blood sugar patients often feel lightheaded and exhausted. They sometimes lose consciousness if the starvation of the brain is severe enough. Palpitation of the heart followed by convulsions has been reported.

Many physicians believe that most alcoholics suffer from hypoglycemia. Some alcoholics report that their doctors have told them to eat candy or some other food high in sugar when they felt they must have liquor. It apparently never occurred to these doctors that when sugar is taken into the body, it must be converted to alcohol before it can be absorbed. So we find "recovered alcoholics" substituting sugar for alcohol and not understanding why they continue to crave liquor.

The physical craving for liquor will continue as long as the alcoholic keeps his chemical merry-go-round in motion, whether from alcohol, sugar, or some other quickly absorbed carbohydrate, and he will feel miserable most of the time.

Undoubtedly there have been more mistakes made in diagnosing the ailments of low blood sugar sufferers than of any other group of ill people. They have been operated on and treated for about every disease on record. Since all such treatments for hypoglycemia are ineffective, there has always been the "hysteria" or the "neurosis" diagnosis to fall back on.

This is the proper diet usually followed for low blood sugar:

*Foods Allowed*

All meats, fish, and shellfish

Dairy products: eggs, milk, butter, and cheese; also, margarines, but none with corn oil

Milk between meals; milk, cheese and/or butter (or margarine) and saltines before retiring

All vegetables and fruits not listed below

Salted nuts (excellent between meals)

Dietetic (no sugar) peanut butter

Protein bread

Soybeans and soybean products

Decaffeinated coffee, weak tea, and sugar-free sodas

Saccharin, sodium cyclamate, or calcium cyclamate, as a substitute for sugar

*Foods to Avoid*

Potatoes, corn, macaroni, spaghetti, rice

Pie, cake, pastries, sugar, candies, dates, and raisins

Cola and other sweet soft drinks

Alcohol in all forms

Coffee and strong tea

All hot and cold cereals, except oatmeal occasionally

Having milk, fruit, or nuts between meals is advisable to prevent blood sugar levels from slackening off (as is apt to occur two or three hours after meals).

The importance of adhering to the above diet cannot be overemphasized. Dietary indiscretion will cause a return of the hateful symptoms of low blood sugar. Unless one has made up his mind to stick with this diet until he overcomes his low blood sugar condition, he will be wasting both his doctor's and his own time in starting on the diet, which is, as is evident, an easy one to follow.

Hypoglycemics all know that their common complaints

of fatigue, weakness, depression, insomnia, nervousness, and apprehensiveness are much worse following physical, emotional, or infection-caused stress. Therefore, they must learn to take environmental and emotional stress in stride. They must work out their own routines which help them control their emotions. They must always remember that they can avoid hypoglycemic reactions by eating less at mealtimes and taking snacks between meals and at bedtime. They must never forget that eating candy or any food with sugar is completely out.

Dr. Juan Carlos De Tata, a prominent Hawaiian psychiatrist, in a medical paper, "Research on Relative Hypoglycemic Syndrome," prepared in the summer of 1967 for eventual publication, wrote:

"Hypoglycemia as a syndrome has been related to neurosis and psychosis. Constant appearance of certain symptoms and adherence to certain diets, usually high in carbohydrate and caffeine, point to the diagnosis of relative hypoglycemic syndrome; however, most of these patients are diagnosed as neurotics. Not diminishing the importance of the psychiatric syndrome, this report summarizes some studies done in the mainland about determination of hypoglycemic syndrome by clinical examination, and 6-hours glucose tolerance tests and our own follow-up of 23 patients. Treatment consists of diet, and, where indicated, calcium, atropine and mild tranquilization.

"The writer became interested in hypoglycemia because of personal reasons. During nine months, from July, 1964, until March, 1965, he had been going from one doctor to the other with complaints of headaches, dizziness, threatened faintings, fatigue, sweating, cold hands and feet, and occasional muscle cramps. All kinds of diagnoses had been offered, from suspicion of stomach ulcer to complete study including EEG and skull X-ray. Finally, a 3-hour glucose tolerance test discovered a 3rd hour drop of 30 points from an original 78 mg. fasting blood sugar to 48 mg. in the third hour.

"Coincidentally I was able to read a note on Roche Report, 'Frontiers of Hospital Psychiatry,' (January, 1966) by Dr. Harry M. Salzer. . . . This note concerned neuropsychiatric illness often caused by relative hypoglycemia. . . .

"Dr. Salzer has found that relative hypoglycemia, a drop in blood sugar levels in response to caffeine and a high carbohydrate intake, was a common cause of neuropsychiatric illness. Dr. Salzer pointed out that from a psychiatric standpoint:

"1. The *major symptoms of the syndrome* were depression, insomnia, anxiety, irritability, lack of concentration, crying spells, phobias, forgetfulness, confusion and asocial or antisocial behavior and even suicidal tendencies.

"2. The *major neurological symptoms* were headaches, dizziness, internal and external *tremulousness*, numbness, blurred vision, staggering, faintings or blackouts, and muscular twitching.

"3. The *extensive somatic symptoms* were exhaustion, fatigue, bloating, abdominal spasms, muscle and joint pains, backache, muscle cramps, colitis and convulsions.

"Dr. Salzer also pointed out that since relative hypoglycemia mimics any neuropsychiatric disorder, patients with that syndrome have been incorrectly diagnosed as having such illnesses as schizophrenia, manic depressive psychosis and psychopathic personality. . . . Dr. Salzer indicated that treatment was simple, requiring only strict adherence to a regimen which would include a high protein, low carbohydrate, frequent feedings, caffeine-free diet. . . . A paper with his studies was presented to the American Medical Association convention. (*Journal of the American Medical Association*, January, 1966, vol. 58, no. 1, pp. 12–17.)"

Dr. De Tata then stated concerning the mental health center with which he is associated, "We have at this clinic carried out a very simple research consisting of 23 patients who came for outpatient psychiatric treatment in which we suspected the presence of relative hypoglycemic syndrome. We utilized a very similar diet to the so-called Seale Harris diet, and we were able to bring about a tremendous improvement in those patients who cooperated with the diet. . . . It is also interesting to note that the local people's diet is mostly starchy, consisting of rice and some vegetable products, and they have tremendous difficulty in following a high-protein diet. Also they are reluctant to abandon coffee. However, in the few cases that did follow our diet, they did wonderfully! Increased ingestion of calcium to improve their concomitant hypocalcemia was also recommended. . . . We certainly insist that every patient with emotional upset try to discover if he is not suffering concomitantly from relative hypoglycemia."[*]

The late Dr. Sam E. Roberts, a distinguished oto-

[*] Quotations from Dr. De Tata's paper have been used with his permission.

laryngologist and author, said that if all patients admitted to mental hospitals were regularly examined for hypoglycemia, and if found suffering from that disease were placed on an antihypoglycemia diet, there would be no shortage of beds in our mental institutions.

Dr. Alan A. Cott, a practicing psychiatrist, estimates that as many as 80 to 90 per cent of schizophrenic patients may suffer from relative hypoglycemia, if not the chronic condition.

Cecilia Rosenfeld, M.D., found in her practice that a surprisingly large number of broken marriages resulted from a blood sugar imbalance in husbands and wives. Dr. Rosenfeld said that when the sugar imbalance was corrected, the emotional stress usually disappeared, and marriage harmony was restored.

Dr. Robert L. Meiers, a psychiatrist of Stanford University Medical School, treats schizophrenia patients for hypoglycemia when that condition exists.

Dr. John W. Tintera, noted New York endocrinologist, has estimated that 80 per cent of those in mental hospitals in America are victims of hypoglycemia.

Dr. Harry M. Salzer, the famous Ohio physician quoted above, reports that he has seen hundreds of patients suffering so severely from hypoglycemia that many of them had been hospitalized in mental institutions.

The distinguished English psychiatrist, Dr. Charles Mercier, aroused Freud's anger by referring to his (Freud's) work as "Freudian fairy tales." Dr. Mercier found many mentally unbalanced people whose mental illnesses were caused by diets too high in starch and sugar and too low in meat. He obtained sensational cures of these people by having them cut down on starch and sugar and eat more meat.

An article appearing in the *Chicago Daily News* on February 25, 1966, reported that the Executive Director of the National Association for Retarded Children believed that a fourth of the children in the United States who were diagnosed as mentally retarded have normal mental abilities.

Dr. Joseph Wilder, of New York, specialist in psychiatry and neurology, found that low blood sugar is far more serious with children than it is with adults. Dr. Wilder said, "The importance of nutrition for mental functioning is much greater in children than in adults. In adults, faulty or insufficient nutrition may alter or impair specific or general mental functions, and eventually cause reparable or even irreparable structural damage of the central nervous system. In children, we face a grave additional factor. The development of the brain may be retarded, stopped, altered, and thus the mental functions may become impaired in indirect and not less serious ways. . . . The child may be neurotic, psychopathic, and be subject to anxiety, running away tendencies, aggressiveness, a blind urge to activity and destructiveness, with impairment of moral sensibilities. . . . In its simplest form, it is a tendency to deny everything, contradict everything, refuse everything, at any price."

Dr. Nicholas R. Occhino, specialist in internal medicine, writing in the October, 1965, issue of *Nutritional Reviews*, described persons suffering from symptoms of mental illness who were returned to health mentally by having been placed on a diet that resulted in normal blood sugar.

He noted that inborn errors of metabolism resulting in mental disorders can sometimes be corrected by the right nutritional program.

The tests for hypoglycemia, or low blood sugar, are neither complicated nor expensive. Most physicians require a thorough endocrine history and a physical examination before making the tests, which consist of:

1. A glucose tolerance test
2. A complete blood count
3. A protein bound iodine test
4. A urine analysis

Some doctors insist on a more elaborate series of laboratory tests; however most physicians agree that the minimal testing shown above is adequate.

One with low blood sugar should not be frightened at having to eliminate foods to which he is accustomed. Dietetic departments of supermarkets, health food stores, and drugstores carry artificially sweetened syrups, jellies, and preserves as tasty as those containing sugar. The permitted diet includes nearly all kinds of fruit and vegetables (without sugar) and all kinds of meats, fish, poultry, and other protein foods.

To help those who are not accustomed to planning meals on a low carbohydrate (slowly absorbed), high protein, and medium fat diet, these menus are given:

## SUGGESTED MENU—
### INEXPENSIVE

*On arising in the morning*

   Fruit juice not sweetened with sugar

*Breakfast*

> One thin slice toasted protein bread with butter or margarine and dietetic jelly
> Fresh fruit, or canned fruit artificially sweetened
> One egg—boiled, poached, scrambled, or fried
> Decaffeinated coffee

*Midmorning snack*

> Cheese (any kind) with 2 or 3 saltines

*Lunch*

> Egg and cheese sandwich (open-face) made with one slice of toasted protein bread; butter or margarine (not corn oil) optional
> Sliced tomatoes
> Serving of cooked vegetable
> Molded gelatin dessert with or without artificially sweetened mixed fruits
> Milk or bone meal tablets

*Midafternoon snack*

> Salted nuts or dietetic peanut butter rolled up in a leaf of lettuce

*Dinner*

> Mixed green vegetable salad with small amount of French or mayonnaise dressing
> Hamburger steak
> Serving of cooked vegetable
> Any permitted fruit for dessert
> Decaffeinated coffee

*Bedtime snack*

> Glass of milk and one thin slice of protein bread or 2 or 3 saltines

## SUGGESTED MENU—
### MORE EXPENSIVE

*On arising in the morning*

> Fruit juice not sweetened with sugar

*Breakfast*

> Ham or sausage and one egg
>
> One thin slice protein bread, toasted if desired, with butter or margarine
>
> Fruit, such as half-grapefruit, orange, nonsweetened applesauce, or any other fruit not excluded from diet
>
> Decaffeinated coffee

*Midmorning snack*

> Milk or dietetic peanut butter and 2 or 3 saltines

*Lunch*

> Grated carrot and cabbage or lettuce salad
>
> Chicken or fish
>
> Cooked vegetable
>
> One slice of protein bread (toasted if desired) with butter or margarine
>
> Melon, any kind

*Midafternoon snack*

> Salted nuts

*Dinner*

> Cottage cheese salad
> Pork chops or lamb chops
> Cooked vegetable
> Cooked dried fruit or fresh fruit
> Decaffeinated coffee

*Bedtime snack*

> Glass of milk and some permitted fruit

## SUGGESTED MENU—
MORE EXPENSIVE

*On arising in the morning*

> Fruit juice not sweetened with sugar

*Breakfast*

> Bacon and two eggs
> One thin slice protein bread (may be toasted) with butter or margarine and artificially sweetened fruit preserves
> Half-grapefruit, half-cantaloupe, or any kind of permitted fruit
> Decaffeinated coffee

*Midmorning snack*

> Glass of milk and 2 or 3 saltines

*Lunch*

> Cottage cheese salad with avocado or unsweetened pineapple
> Ham, ground steak, fish, or fowl

One cooked vegetable

One slice of protein bread (toasted if desired) with butter or margarine

*Midafternoon snack*

Salted nuts

*Dinner*

Tossed green salad with or without small amount of French or mayonnaise dressing

Roast beef or steak, the latter perferably broiled

One cooked vegetable

Dietetic ice cream

Decaffeinated coffee

*Bedtime snack*

Glass of milk with thin slice of protein bread or dietetic peanut butter and 2 or 3 saltines

# 4
# Vitamins bring
# mental health

The antagonism of many physicians to nutrition as a means of obtaining and keeping mental health is well known. It would seem that the great expense and too frequent futility of psychoanalysis would have driven the psychiatrists to a study of nutrition as a possible aid in helping the mentally disturbed. It is true that the tranquilizers have, to some extent, replaced the long hours of couch therapy, but the most ardent advocates of tranquilizing drugs will not contend that they cure those to whom they are administered.

Ancel Keys and his associates conducted a series of tests on a group for 120 days, during which time both physiological and psychological tests were made almost daily. The results were described in the book *Biology of Human Starvation*, published in 1950 by the University of Minnesota Press. This study of starvation as a cause of mental illness was conducted by the Laboratory of Physiological Hygiene, School of Public Health of the University of Minnesota.

The report showed that nutritional privation caused psychoneurosis, and that there is no basic difference between the responses of a normal volunteer suffering from nutritional privation and mental patients diagnosed as such by psychiatrists.

Again, in 1954, R. A. Peterman and R. S. Goodhart, reporting in the *Journal of Clinical Nutrition*, had induced a number of apparent mental disorders among subjects deprived of specific vitamins. To be more exact, they found that a lack of thiamine brought ideas of persecution, mental confusion, and bad memory; a deficiency of riboflavin caused depression, visual disturbances, disordered thinking, and inability to concentrate; not enough niacin resulted in unreasonable fears, anxiety, mania, hallucinations and dementia; insufficient pyridoxine produced convulsions, irritability, and general weakness.

In 1954, as reported in the *Journal of Psychology*, G. Watson and A. L. Comrey conducted a study to determine the value of vitamins and minerals in two groups, one given placebos and the others a multiple-vitamin formula. The results so conclusively showed the value of vitamins and the worthlessness of placebos that the researchers determined that, in some cases, mental illness, as diagnosed by psychiatrists, can be relieved by nutritional means.

George Watson, in 1954 in the *Journal of Psychology*, tells how a mentally disturbed girl with suicidal tendencies, a feeling of revulsion toward her father, and fear of leaving her room, was cured in a relatively short time by correct nutrition.

Watson believes that subjects who are beginning to feel the effect of nutritional stress and who are upset emotionally, and sometimes also their doctors, make the mistake of looking for the cause of their troubles in their relationships with others. He says, "Instead of saying, 'I am upset, what is wrong with my body chemistry?' they are apt to say, 'I am upset. What did you do to me, and why did you do it?' "

Dr. Humphry Osmond, famed psychiatrist, has explained why physicians generally have been indifferent to nutrition as a means of helping the mentally ill. "Medical men," said Dr. Osmond, "are often inclined to think of vitamins in minute doses. The curative effect of large doses of vitamins is foreign to their thinking."

Dr. A. A. Pokrovsky, director of the Institute of Nutrition of the U.S.S.R. National Academy of Medical Sciences, speaking recently at an International Conference on Malnutrition, Learning, and Behavior at the Massachusetts Institute of Technology, stated: "There is no doubt protein is important, but protein is not the only nutrient affecting mental development, nor is it the only one of which malnourished children fail to get enough. . . . And even though not every nutrient is directly involved in the development of the nervous system, malnutrition of any type will cause malfunctioning of the metabolism and that will affect the health and abilities of the brain." Dr. Pokrovsky went on to name niacin (vitamin $B_3$) as likely being deficient in the diets of children whose mental functions do not develop properly.

It has only been for the last few years that we have understood how the foods we put into our stomachs control the quality of our mental abilities. We now know why it is so important to our mental health to have a steady, daily supply of the highest quality protein, containing the right amino acids.

Recently, an eminent nutritionist, Dr. David Coursin, in discussing the relationship between nutrition and mentality, at the Massachusetts Institute of Technology, named every single vitamin of the B complex, as well as vitamins A and C, as "particularly important to central nervous system activity." Dr. Coursin spoke of deficiencies in any of these vitamins in early childhood as leading to irreversible harmful effects on the nervous system, or what we ordinarily call mental retardation.

Dr. Joan Caddell, of the George Washington School of Medicine, reported in the October 1, 1966, issue of *The Lancet* that children appearing to have mental apathy and depression, loss of coordination, and decreased strength, probably had a mineral (magnesium) deficiency as well as a vitamin (thiamine) deficiency.

Physicians have known for years that vitamin A increases longevity and delays senility. Discoveries are being made so rapidly of the healing properties of all the vitamins that we may expect some dramatic revelations to be made by members of the medical profession almost daily.

Since half of the patients in our mental hospitals have been diagnosed as suffering from schizophrenia, heretofore considered incurable, separate chapters of this book will be devoted to discussing this awful disease and what has been accomplished in overcoming it.

The problem of declining mental abilities for the aged has baffled doctors for generations. Most physicians have accepted confusion, disorientation, and failure of memory as something that inevitably comes with age. More advanced-thinking doctors have recognized these conditions as resulting from starved cells of the brain, but knowing no alternative, have accepted the situation with resignation.

Drs. Franklin I. Shuman and Ronald I. Goldberg, of the New England Hospital (Boston), used a successful therapy in restoring the mentalities of elderly patients. As published in the June, 1965, issue of the *Journal of the American Geriatric Society*, these physicians obtained good results in 66 per cent of patients with enfeebled minds, fair results with 25 per cent, and poor results with 9 per cent.

The basis of the treatment was nicotinic acid (now generally called niacin), vitamin $B_3$, in combination with high-potency multivitamin supplements. Drs. Shuman and Goldberg said in their report, "The geriatric patient is prone to use an abnormal diet (e.g., soup and crackers) and as such is subject to the development of vitamin deficiencies. It is therefore important that any therapeutic agent for the treatment of senility should contain a high-potency preparation." These doctors point out that the answer is some therapy that retards the aging process— or, put in layman's language, a diet that contains the essential vitamins (particularly niacin, or vitamin $B_3$) — *before* one reaches a senile condition.

Dr. William Sargent, an English psychiatrist, writing in a late issue of *The Atlantic Monthly*, said: "Most psychiatrists visiting the United States from abroad are bewildered by the way the direction and control of American psychiatry have been taken over since World War II by psychoanalysts who are ideological followers of Freud . . . a state of affairs which prevails in no other country in the world at the present time. It has generally been found over the years that psychoanalysis is a poor weapon to treat most forms of mental and even neurotic illness. One has only to go today into the mental hospitals in the United States to see the total failure of Freudian methods."

German physicians in the Max-Planck Institute for Medical Research in Heidelberg have found that vitamin $B_6$ (pyridoxine) reduces fatigue, headache, insomnia, inability to concentrate, loss of memory, and general decline of intelligence. However, the *German Tribune*, December 21, 1963, quoted Dr. Birkmayer, a Vienna neurologist, speaking before the Neurology Congress in Augsburg, as warning against the indiscriminate use of pyridoxine as a wonder drug for mental ailments. Other nutritionists have warned that any one of the B-complex vitamins, taken separately, may create an imbalance presenting a real danger to one experimenting with such vitamins. *No single B vitamin should ever be used except under the supervision of a physician.*

Dr. David Coursin reported in a 1954 issue of the *Journal of the American Medical Association* that he gave a dosage of 100 mgs. of pyridoxine (vitamin $B_6$) intramuscularly to one hundred patients with various illnesses related to the central nervous system, with spectacular results, especially in patients with brain disorders.

As early as 1939, researchers reported in the *Bulletin of the Staff of the Mayo Clinic* (vol. 14, p. 787) on an experiment with patients deprived of thiamine (vitamin $B_1$) for ten days to five weeks. They became confused, uncertain of memory, irritable, depressed, quarrelsome, uncooperative, and fearful of impending disaster.

Dr. Tom Spies, in 1943, in the *Association for Research on Nervous Disorders* (vol. 22, p. 122), told of 115 patients eating a diet low in thiamine. They became timid and depressed people, but within thirty minutes to twenty hours after receiving supplementary vitamin $B_1$ they became pleasant and cooperative.

In the chapter "Nutrition in Disease" in *The Heinz Handbook of Nutrition* (2nd ed.), it is stated: "Thiamine deficiency is considered responsible for the peripheral nerve degeneration and central nervous system changes found in long-standing cases of chronic alcoholism." The author goes on to list these central nervous system changes resulting from a lack of thiamine, "personality changes, hallucinosis and amnesia."

Dr. M. Calvario reported in 1958 in an Italian publication, *Acia Vitaminologica*, that he had made complete studies between pyridoxine (vitamin $B_6$) deficiencies and epileptic convulsions. With the administration of this vitamin, forty epileptic patients were helped.

Drs. W. W. Umbriet and J. Waddell, discoverers of pyridoxine in 1949, carried out experiments with volunteers to determine what happened when this vitamin was destroyed. The subjects responded with malfunctions of the central nervous system, including convulsions.

In the June 27, 1959, *Journal of the American Medical Association* the story is related of a forty-four-year-old housewife who was admitted to a mental hospital on a diagnosis of severe mental breakdown. She had hallucinations and delusions. Intramuscular injection of vitamin $B_{12}$ quickly restored mental balance.

Dr. J. G. Henderson, a psychiatrist at the University of Aberdeen, wrote in *The Lancet* for October 16, 1966: "The psychiatrist must expect to encounter the mental illness of vitamin $B_{12}$ deficiency in patients who have neither anemia nor any evidence of subacute combined degeneration of the cord. Moreover, since the mental disorder of vitamin $B_{12}$ is protean in character, and can even occur in childhood, it is a possible diagnosis in the majority of psychiatric patients."

This statement is found in the *Journal of the American Medical Association* for June 27, 1959: "Mental changes resulting from vitamin $B_{12}$ deficiency are among the least publicized aspects of this condition. The cerebral manifestations of this disorder have received little consideration in standard textbooks on the subject. The milder symptoms may be a slight mood disturbance or mental slowness with difficulty in concentrating and remembering. The symptoms may be much more severe, however, with violent maniacal behavior, severe agitation, stuperous depression, paranoid behavior, or the presence of overt visual and auditory hallucinations. . . . When present, these mental status findings make it difficult to distinguish this condition from schizophrenia."

This statement is from the *British Medical Journal* of March 26, 1966: "It is true that vitamin $B_{12}$ deficiency may cause severe psychotic symptoms which may vary in severity from mild disorders of mood, mental slowness, and memory defect to severe psychotic symptoms including agitation, depression, severe confusional and hallucinatory states, and paranoid behavior. Occasionally these mental disturbances may be the first manifestations of $B_{12}$ deficiency."

Dr. Michael Jefferson, a British neurologist, said in *The Practitioner*, January, 1964, that simple vitamin B deficiency is responsible for many of the complaints of middle age. He also mentioned that the B vitamins are all of special importance to the proper functioning of the nervous system.

Dr. Jefferson further stated that vitamin $B_{12}$ needs may show up in lack of attentiveness, forgetfulness, disorientation, and mood changes. In the elderly, this may be mistaken for senility or psychosis. "In a few cases there is a dramatic response to treatment, so that symptoms and signs of nervous dysfunction resolve in a few weeks; but in the majority, their warning is slow and it is likely to be six or twelve months before dimensions of residual disability can be fully assessed," Dr. Jefferson wrote.

The *American Journal of Psychiatry* carried an article in August, 1965, to the effect that heavy doses of niacin included in daily multiple-vitamin therapy had eliminated cases of dizziness, headaches, and nervousness of twenty years' duration.

The famous nutritionist Norman Jolliffe has observed: "Almost every vitamin has been credited with playing a role in the maintenance of a normal nervous system. The more important of the vitamins thus accredited are thiamin hydrochloride, nicotinic acid, riboflavin, pyridoxine and alpha-tocopherol."

*The Lancet* for October 9, 1965, has an article by Drs. Richard Hunter and D. M. Matthews, psychiatrists, showing that vitamin $B_{12}$ deficiency may precede any outward signs of mental illness by days or months, and that a wide variety of mental illnesses have a vitamin $B_{12}$ deficiency at their root. These doctors suggested that a $B_{12}$ deficiency screening became routine among psychiatric patients.

*The Lancet* for January 7, 1967, quoted several English physicians as having recommended that every mental patient who had gastric surgery should be tested for vitamin $B_{12}$ deficiency. Twenty English mental patients who had had parts of their stomachs removed were studied. Five had vitamin $B_{12}$ deficiency which caused their mental illnesses. Two others had vitamin $B_{12}$ insufficiency which contributed to their mental troubles. Two were found to be deficient in iron.

The New York *Herald Tribune* on February 17, 1959, quoted the highly respected Dr. Victor Herbert, of New York's Mt. Sinai Hospital, as placing the blame for many patients being committed to mental hospitals on brain damage resulting from a lack of $B_{12}$ vitamin.

*The New York Times* on April 20, 1968, discussed a report by Dr. Linus Pauling, twice Nobel Prize-winning chemist from the University of California at San Diego, in which Dr. Pauling cited recent research to support his belief that the brain and nervous system may be especially affected by deficiencies in vitamins and other chemical substances. Human beings, he said, may be subject to a sort of "cerebral scurvy or cerebral pernicious anemia."

To support his argument, the California scientist cited cases in which vitamin $B_{12}$ seemed to play a part in mental illness. "A low concentration of $B_{12}$ in the blood has been reported to occur for a much larger proportion of patients with mental illness than for the general population," said Dr. Pauling, who stated that he associated vitamin C, thiamine, folic acid, and glutamic acid deficiencies with mental illness.

In the same issue of *The New York Times* is a report by Dr. Stephan Zamenhoff and other biochemists of the University of California in Los Angeles, showing that tests made on laboratory animals whose mothers were deficient in protein during pregnancy indicated mental impairment in the offspring. The scientists who made the studies said their findings may explain "the impaired behavior and learning ability in children of malnourished mothers."

Drs. Smith and Oliver related in the *British Medical Journal* of July 1, 1967, the story of a woman who apparently was well nourished, but depressed. Four days after entering the hospital, she became confused, had delusions and hallucinations, and could be kept in the hospital only while tranquilized. She was given injections of vitamin $B_{12}$ and within twenty-four hours her mental condition started improving, and within a few days her mental symptoms were normal.

Another article, appearing in the *British Medical Journal* for July 23, 1966, showed that researchers found that 67 per cent of aged hospitalized persons, unable to take care of themselves and considered as mental patients, were deficient in folic acid, one of the B vitamins. This vitamin deficiency was traced to dietary habits, or simple malnutrition.

Dr. H. Grabner wrote in the October 31, 1958, *Münchener Medizinische Wochenschrift* that he had experimented with patients considered beyond the hope of any treatment. He became convinced that vitamin $B_{12}$ therapy could be used successfully in various neurological and psychiatric cases, including polio and muscular dystrophy, epilepsy, and schizophrenia.

The *British Medical Journal* of May 10, 1958, told about a seventy-one-year-old man who had seldom been ill. Called on to treat an arthritic complaint, the physician found his patient in bed in such a state of mental confusion that he spoke incoherently, was unable to find or use the lavatory, and could not dress himself. Only vitamin B was prescribed, and in a month the man had fully recovered. Without consulting his doctor, the patient discontinued the vitamin B treatment and suffered a relapse into his former condition. When vitamin B was again used, he was back to normal in a week.

Dr. P. Berkenau, of the English Warneford Hospital, said, in an article in the *Journal of Mental Science* (vol. 86, p. 675), that he had tested a group of senile patients, along with another group who were mentally alert. He added fairly large amounts of ascorbic acid (vitamin C) to the daily diet of each. His belief was that those with vitamin C in their tissues would require less time to reach the absorption point than those deficient in vitamin C. (Dr. Berkenau demonstrated that all the senile patients were deficient in vitamin C, whereas the normal patients showed little or no lack of this vitamin.) Dr. Berkenau said that a deficit of 1,000 to 1,500 mgs. of vitamin may be regarded as pathological, whereas his tests showed that the senile oldsters tested had shortages of from 2,400 to 3,000 mgs. of vitamin C.

Dr. C. Milner wrote in the *British Journal of Psychiatry* that he had tested the blood of forty mentally ill patients for ascorbic acid content. Each one had a definite vitamin C shortage. Then, for three weeks, each patient received 1,000 mgs. of ascorbic acid daily. All of them showed significant improvement in the depressive manic and paranoid symptoms. It normally takes only twenty-four to forty-eight hours to saturate the tissues of a normal patient with ascorbic acid; it took an average of six days to saturate the tissues of the abnormally acting patients. "Psychiatric patients," said Dr. Milner, "are shown to have an unusually high demand for ascorbic acid."

Dr. Roger J. Williams, of the University of Texas, told the National Academy of Sciences, on April 27, 1967, that vitamin C requirements in individuals vary too much to rely on blanket recommendations. Dr. Williams based his conclusions on the vitamin C requirements of guinea pigs. Some got along quite well on small amounts; others required much more vitamin C.

The spring (1964) issue of the British *Clinical Physiology* carries the report of a study of forty psychiatric patients whose tissues were saturated with vitamin C, after which all showed improvement. It was therefore concluded that psychiatric patients have a high demand for ascorbic acid.

Dr. Evan Shute, world's foremost authority on vitamin E, noted in his book *Alpha Tocopherol in Cardiovascular Disease* that degenerative diseases, the plague of modern civilization, may be the result of long-time partial vitamin E deficiency. Dr. Shute continues, "It may well be that the administration of adequate alpha tocopherol (vitamin E) from infancy onward could retard the onset of the aging process, permitting men to attain a much more advanced and healthful age than is either possible or likely now."

Dr. Aloys Tappel, biochemist at the University of California, recently said, "Aging is due to the process of oxidation, and since vitamin E is a natural anti-oxidant, it could be used to counteract this process in the body."

Dr. Tom Spies, previously referred to, has found that some forms of nervousness respond favorably to vitamin E therapy.

The November, 1964, issue of the *American Journal of Mental Deficiency* discussed many test cases where vitamin E (sometimes with vitamin C) has been given mentally retarded children, generally with beneficial results.

Herbert Bailey, noted science writer and author of the book *Vitamin E: Your Key to a Healthy Heart*, pointed out that vitamin E plays an important part in preventing the symptoms of old age.

Dr. Hans Selye and associates have conclusively shown that rats fed massive doses of vitamin E showed no signs of aging and that "old" rats fed vitamin E actually showed a reversal of the aging process.

This word comes from the *Journal of the American Geriatrics Society* for October, 1967: "The prematurely old, those who look old though middle-aged or younger, are apparently suffering from protein, electrolyte, hor-

mone, enzyme and vitamin deficiencies caused by mal-
absorption from the intestinal tract. Hungarian researchers
conclude that 'chronic malnutrition may cause premature
old age.' "

The need for vitamin and mineral nourishment, not
only for the body, but also for the brain, continues from
the cradle to the grave.

A group of Indonesian researchers, led by Drs. Tjiook
Tiauw Hie, Oey Henk Jan, and Lauw Tjin Giok, using
tests given by the psychology faculty of the University
of Indonesia, examined 107 children of from five to twelve
years old. Their report, which appeared in the December,
1967, *American Journal of Clinical Nutrition*, showed a
very low grade of intelligence in the group which had
symptoms of vitamin A deficiency and other indications of
malnutrition. Children with symptoms of vitamin A deficiency were the most mentally retarded.

Drs. Reba Hill and Leighton Hill, of the Pediatrics
Department of Baylor University, had an interesting
report in the December 18, 1967, *Medical Tribune*. They
found that malnourished infants fall behind in mental
development and are subject to neurological disorders.
The study, made over a three-year period, was of 55 infants whose parents were middle-class and 90 per cent
of whom were high school graduates. "In other words,"
commented the Drs. Hill, "these infants were not malnourished or small because of neglect or inadequate
medical care by ignorant parents."

Dr. Geron Churchill, of the Neurology Department at
Detroit Lafayette Clinic, found that mothers whose children have abnormally low IQ's admit poor diets during

pregnancy. "They tended to eat nothing all day but crackers and soda pop; they'd have a big meal at night when their husbands came home. . . . Many times I found their diets were top-heavy with carbohydrates and far too low in protein. It's odd in a privileged population such as we have today, when so much good nutrition is available. These women weren't poor." Dr. Churchill continued: "A very delicate balance for particular nutrients is needed during pregnancy. If this balance is upset for periods of time, it appears that the baby's brain may not be completed."

Dr. Pearl Swanson, professor of nutrition at Iowa State University, has continually reminded us that there is no reason for aging to be synonymous with poor health. She said, "Older people have not lost their capacity to build new tissue . . . when their diets provide adequate protein, calcium and vitamin D. Aging persons will react positively to dietary improvement."

Dr. Swanson found that after thirty the daily intake of calcium usually goes down steadily and that many oldsters were getting only a fourth of the recommended calcium allowance. The B and C vitamins required fell into the same category of neglect.

Two Hungarian physicians, Drs. M. Vass and L. Acs, investigated the nutritional habits of 86 elderly patients. They found a shortage of vitamins to be common with these people. They also found that 64.7 per cent were calcium-deficient. The most important part of their report was that it took vitamin A in high doses to bring the calcium level up. We have been taught for years that vitamin D is necessary for utilization of calcium, and we know of no findings to the contrary, but these Hungarian doctors reported that with old persons vitamin A, when administered in doses three times as high as the ordinary daily requirement of a healthy adult, would bring up the blood calcium level.

In the October, 1967, *Journal of the American Geriatrics Society*, Dr. Susana Dennes reported the case of Mrs. S. B., a 43-year-old disability pensioner, who looked 60 and whose tests showed that her body functioned like that of a 60-year-old woman. Here was a textbook case of premature old age due to poor nutritional choices in eating.

When we hear doctors come into court and testify that senility is inevitable with advanced age, we know they are not willfully committing perjury. We know that is what they believe because that is what they were taught in medical school. No informed student of nutrition believes that old age and senility have to march together.

For at least thirty years, American physicians have known that vitamin deficiencies can and do cause neurologic and psychiatric disorders. We shall briefly discuss a few of the physical diseases with apparent mental disorganization and confusion that have successfully responded to vitamin therapy.

*Pellagra*

Numerous isolated cases of pellagra were reported in the United States before 1906, and since then the disease increased, but no effective cure was found until 1938, when several workers in various parts of the nation reported excellent results with nicotinic acid (niacin), one of the B vitamins, in the treatment of pellagra.

Later, doctors discovered that pellagra sufferers were also deficient in other members of the B complex, especially thiamine, riboflavin, and pyridoxine. Niacin ($B_3$) alone dramatically relieved the early mental syndrome of pellagra, but with the neurological damage in long-standing cases all B vitamins and multivitamin supplemental feeding must be given, so researchers have found.

The early signs of this disease are irritability, headaches, and emotional instability. In later stages, loss of memory, confusional psychosis with hallucinations, delirium, and apparent schizophrenia are observed. Some of the patients with advanced pellagra have cogwheel rigidity of the extremities, and at times coma is present.

Massive doses of niacin are usually given by "shots" in the bloodstream for a few days, then oral administration of huge doses of niacin and other vitamin supplements are followed for some time. A high protein diet of liver, eggs, milk, and meat is always indicated for the pellagra patient.

When vitamin therapy was first suggested for pellagra, doctors were as much against using it as are some doctors now who oppose the use of vitamins, minerals, and other nutrients with patients who, according to these physicians, have only "diseases of the psyche." At one time 10 per cent of the patients admitted to mental hospitals in the southern part of the nation had pellagra but were diagnosed as schizophrenics.

Postmortems on advanced pellagra patients have shown general tissue degeneration. Others have been found to have a curious mummified bodily condition. Some scientists believe that pellagra may be of a diabetic origin.

### Beriberi

This disease is still common in Southeast Asia, although some cases are found in America. It is prevalent among poor people who live mostly on a carbohydrate diet.

In 1890, Dr. Charles Hose, after studying the eating habits in Sarawak, became convinced that beriberi had some connection with diet. In 1911, the great biochemist Casimir Funk fractionated rice polishings and obtained a crystalline product, for which he coined the term "vitamine." Jansen and Donath (1926) were the first to isolate a single substance from a natural source which had a curative effect on beriberi. Williams and Cline, in 1936, reported the synthesis of a crystalline material which they called "thiamine."

Some of the neurological symptoms of advanced beriberi are extreme nervousness, decreased perception of touch, double vision, loss of memory, confusion, hallucinations, and, in extreme cases, stupor and coma.

Beriberi responds favorably to massive doses of thiamine (vitamin $B_1$) and a generous supply of high-quality proteins.

### Scurvy

This is perhaps the oldest of the known vitamin-deficiency diseases; history tells us that in 1795 the regulated use of lime juice was begun in the British navy in order to cure and prevent scurvy of sailors. Disorders of vision, profound exhaustion, and general mental confusion go with scurvy.

Scurvy readily responds to ascorbic acid (vitamin C)

and a diet rich in certain fruits and vegetables high in vitamin C.

### Wernicke's Encephalopathy

This degenerative disease of the brain, characterized by double vision, muscular incoordination, loss of memory, confusion, and hallucinations, is the result of thiamine (vitamin $B_1$) deficiency. Massive doses of thiamine and a high-caloric, high-protein and moderate-fat diet are prescribed.

### Kwashiorkor

Kwashiorkor is a protein-calorie nutritional disease, usually of infancy and early childhood, although some adults have the disease. It is widely prevalent among the poor in Africa, India, Central and South America, the West Indies, Mexico, and Southeast Asia.

The disease results from a diet consisting largely of starchy paps and a consequent failure to provide proteins. Infants and children with kwashiorkor are frequently considered to be feebleminded, but after multiple-vitamin, high-protein, medium-carbohydrate, and mineral feedings, if and when they recover from the disease they are found to have normal minds.

There are several other vitamin-deficiency diseases, such as avitaminosis A, a vitamin-A-deficiency disease; rickets, a vitamin-D-deficiency disease; and ariboflavinosis, a riboflavin (vitamin $B_2$)-deficiency disease.

We have discussed these vitamin-deficiency diseases to show how the normal functioning of the human organ system and tissues, and of the peripheral and central nervous systems, are dependent on a nutrition that includes adequate vitamins. It has also been our purpose to explain that the administration of vitamins for the relief of physical diseases that have abnormal mental manifestations is not new to the medical profession.

# 5

# Schizophrenia,
# a physical disease
# that affects the mind

Schizophrenia is understood by most physicians and laymen to be a mental disease. Bleuler said that dementia praecox, or mental deterioration characterized by disorientation, loss of contact with reality, and splitting of the personality, is the same as schizophrenia. The difficulty with medical definitions of schizophrenia usually is that they were formulated by disciples of Sigmund Freud, who was fascinated by hypnotism, obsessed by sex, and in his writings indicated that he was himself suffering from psychoneurosis.

Dr. Robert S. de Ropp, a biochemist, in his book *Drugs and the Mind*, tells us about two schizophrenics. The first one is Mary, twenty-eight years old, institutionalized for eight years. "We find her huddled in a corner of a wooden bench, completely motionless, her knees drawn up under her chin and her thin arms clasped about her legs. Her short, cropped hair is in disorder, her body so thin that the bones are visible through the flesh. She is wearing nothing but a shabby nightgown made of a heavy coarse material, for in her occasional fits of violence she is liable to strip off her clothing and tear it to pieces.

§71

"Most of the time, however, she remains motionless, not moving even to satisfy the calls of nature or to take food. If you move her arm, it remains in any position in which you happen to place it. . . . As she will not eat, food has to be introduced into her stomach. As she will not attend to her needs, she has to be changed like a baby.

"The attendants have come to regard her as virtually an inanimate object, like a piece of furniture. . . . All her contacts with the outer world have been severed. Her husband has moved to a state in which insanity constitutes valid grounds for divorce, has freed himself from the burden, and married again. Her children do not remember her.

"Her illness began when she was twenty. She may live on into her sixties. For all those forty years she must be cared for—a living corpse denied even the privilege of burial."

About George, the other schizophrenic, Dr. de Ropp writes:

"He is about the same age as Mary, but does not sit motionless as she does. George, in fact, is very active, but his activity has no connection with the realities of this world, for within the labyrinth of George's mind is a distorting mirror which prevents even the simplest impression from reaching his brain unaltered.

"Everything he sees, everything he hears, the things he touches, the food he eats, becomes endowed, through the action of this distorting agent, with sinister, malignant significance. The words of one of the physicians, the glance of an attendant, even a casual gesture by one of his fellow inmates, is interpreted as a threat.

"The radio broadcasts the plottings of some foreign power disguised to resemble ordinary news or music. The scent of a flower is really a poisoned gas being secretly brewed by 'the enemy' under the floor boards. Often his food has a strange metallic taste. Again it is 'the enemy' attempting to poison him.

"He pushes the food away and refuses to eat for several days. When they try to feed him by force, he fights and screams and struggles, knowing that he has fallen into the hands of 'the enemy,' and that they are about to kill him. Like Mary, he may live for another forty years, alone as only the mad can be alone, a curse to himself, a burden to those who must care for him."

Cases like Mary and George are found in the back wards of all our large mental hospitals where, as Dr. de Ropp so vividly states, behind locked doors, the more violently disturbed patients pass their lives, often herded together under conditions which should be judged unsuitable even for animals.

"For every totally disabled inmate of a mental hospital," says Dr. de Ropp, "at least two others are living in the outer world, not sick enough to be institutionalized, not well enough to live healthy, happy lives. This huge population of mentally sick individuals imposes a burden on the healthy segment of the population whose size is appalling to contemplate. In terms of cost, no other form of illness is more expensive. In terms of suffering, no other affliction is more devastating."●

One of the tragic things about any mental illness is the anguish it produces among the parents, spouses, brothers,

● With permission from St. Martin's Press, New York, © 1957.

sisters, and children of its victims. It has been estimated that one out of three families in America is in some way involved with mental illness. Lawrence Galton, writing in *The New York Times* on November 6, 1966, estimated that two million people in the United States and Canada suffer from schizophrenia.

The recovery rate for schizophrenics has been low and the rate of readmissions to hospitals has been high. Because patients have not received the most advanced treatments, or have been given no treatment at all, the number of readmissions of schizophrenics to mental hospitals is almost equal to the number of first admissions.

It is no wonder that the word "schizophrenia" strikes terror in the hearts of those diagnosed as schizophrenics and their loved ones. The British biologist Sir Julian Huxley has called this disease "the plague of the Twentieth Century."

It is interesting to observe that, notwithstanding the wonderful strides made in medicine on other fronts, the natural recovery rate of schizophrenics has not increased during the past one hundred years. Dr. John Connolly, physician to the Middlesex Asylum in Hanwell, England, noted in 1849 that "the natural course of the disease accounted for the recovery of fifty per cent of the patients."

Every year, thousands of young Americans disappear behind locked doors—the victims of schizophrenia—many of whom will never be heard from again. The loss of so much potential talent and ability is worse than tragic. Physicians and laymen have been so indifferent that not until 1964 was there *one* agency devoted solely to the cause of schizophrenia. In that year the American Schizophrenia Foundation of Ann Arbor, Michigan, was founded. This organization (which we shall hereafter refer to as the Foundation) is carrying out a gigantic task in helping the sufferers of schizophrenia and their families. Much of the information contained in this chapter came from the publications of the Foundation.

The Foundation is also doing a wonderful service to humanity in getting rid of some of the myths and misconceptions surrounding this awful disease. Its constant reminder that *schizophrenia, if diagnosed early and properly treated, is a highly recoverable disease* has brought hope and health to thousands.

The following is a list of important facts about schizophrenia:

1. *Schizophrenia is not caused by the conduct of others.*
How often have we heard it said, "She drove him crazy" or "He drove her out of her mind." People are even ashamed of their schizophrenic relatives and blame the patients for being hospitalized, as if that were their choice of how to live.

Dr. Humphry Osmond says that those suffering from this disease are generally characterized as "comical or pathetic," but never as courageous humans valiantly fighting a disease. Dr. Osmond states that people don't even want to use the word schizophrenia, because it frightens them too much.

Wives or husbands are often blamed for the mental illness of their spouses, thus bringing unwarranted mental anguish to innocent persons. If cancer strikes one's wife or husband or he or she suffers a heart attack, the illness is accepted as a fact of nature, but not so with schizophrenia.

2. *Changing a schizophrenic's environment does not help him.*
Some of the old wives' tales about how these unfortunates can be helped are so ridiculous that it seems preposterous that they would ever have been considered seriously; yet they and many others have been tried. Having a husband leave his wife, separating a child from his parents, and moving away from bothersome neighbors are a few of the silly environmental changes tried—without success.

3. *Schizophrenia is both a physical and psychological disease.* (This will be discussed later.)

4. *Schizophrenia is not a "split" or a "double" personality.*
Notwithstanding the teachings of the idol of many American psychiatrists, Freud, called "the cleverest charlatan the world has even known" by Maurice Natenberg in his book *The Case History of Sigmund Freud*, the dramatic recoveries of schizophrenics in recent years show how false is the myth of the "split," or "double," personality. Natenberg says that even though European psychiatrists have laughed Freud off years ago, Freudian notions still enchant many American writers, newsmen, artists, and intellectuals.

In chapter 2 of his book, Dr. Pinckney tells us that people in the fields of literature, entertainment, child care, education, social welfare, and business have accepted and propagated Freud's theories. Art, too frequently, purports to display the artist's rebellion against the world around him. Sexual symbolism from the unconscious is sought. Psychoanalysis has invaded literature, movies, the theatre, and television with an avalanche of sexual themes.

Without going into detail, the Freudian theme of every conceivable form of immorality and perversion being offered to the public by every possible medium available, is having its effect on our society and its morality. What kind of children and future adults can we expect to come from a generation in which shows, whether on the stage, in motion pictures or by television, dissect perversions, expose man's alleged utter helplessness, and stress the claimed evil in man's nature?

In law enforcement, we frequently find that the Freudian "bleeding hearts" try to take over and excuse murderers, rapists, and other criminals by psychoanalytically placing the blame for their crimes on their parents or society.

The fictional capon of Freud, who has been successively castrated by his mother, his wife and his daughters, is such an unrealistic person that it seems impossible that rational minds would not find such rubbish so revolting and disgusting that they would reject all of Freud's teaching.

The most charitable view we can take of the futile attempts to treat schizophrenics by modern-day psychiatrists who refuse to recognize that their patients are physically ill is that such treatments are more humane than were the beatings of the mentally disturbed administered many, many years ago in the belief that the evil spirits could be driven out of the bodies of the mentally ill by repeated acts of brutality.

5. *Schizophrenia is not a crime or a way of life.*
A popular belief is that schizophrenics are violent murderers. Dr. Osmond says: "While it's true that schizophrenia frequently figures in crime—suicide, homicide, juvenile delinquency, alcoholism and drug addiction—the vast majority of schizophrenics are sensible, harmless, law-abiding citizens enduring a grave and crippling illness."

Lee Harvey Oswald was diagnosed as having had "schizophrenic tendencies" at the age of thirteen. Dr. Osmond says that mental health treatment is so medieval that "had Oswald been treated as most schizophrenics are today, it is doubtful, in my view, whether President Kennedy's life would have been spared. . . . One wonders how long the public will continue to tolerate our bungling, inefficient mental institutions and our Victorian methods of treating schizophrenics." At another time, Dr. Osmond declared, "No one speaks for the schizophrenic, the most helpless and the most afflicted man in the human race."

Again, Dr. Osmond asserted, "Surely, when the public reads about the daily misfortunes which our newspapers are forever attributing to 'a former mental patient,' they are not likely to be persuaded that our institutions are doing an especially good job."

6. *Treatment of schizophrenia by "psychoanalytical" or "psychodynamic" theories does no good, and often aggravates a potentially dangerous condition.*
Too often, despite Freud's explicit warning that schizo-

phrenia does not respond to psychoanalysis, a patient may undergo years of such treatment at tremendous expense. Dr. Robert G. Heath, chairman of the Department of Psychiatry at Tulane University, says it is of the "utmost importance" for a physician to recognize early the presence of schizophrenia, because the therapist who doesn't "may undertake a type of therapy that can result in dire consequences."

Kahlil Samra, president of the Foundation, wrote, in the *Newsletter* of the organization for October, 1967: "One thing we have not done. We have not remained silent about the systematic bilking of patients and their families by practitioners who charge excessive fees for therapies which have been known to be ineffective in the treatment of schizophrenia ever since Clifford Beers founded the N.C.M.H. [National Commission for Mental Hygiene]."

7. *Education regarding the prevalence of schizophrenia and the need for early treatment is urgent.*
The Foundation is trying to keep physicians and clergymen up to date on the latest developments in the diagnosis and treatment of schizophrenia.

Equally important, the Foundation is endeavoring to educate patients and their families as to the nature, extent, and effects of this form of mental illness.

Not only does the A.S.F. (American Schizophrenia Foundation) concern itself with schizophrenics at home, it also strives to ensure hospitalized schizophrenics with the best treatment available consistent with modern medical knowledge. In one of its published bulletins will be found this statement: "Though excellent mental hospitals were designed, built and run in the United States more than a hundred years ago, during the last century standards have fallen deplorably. The sickest schizophrenia patients are often housed under conditions so unsuitable that they increase their chances of remaining permanently ill."

8.   *Schizophrenia is responsible for many of the suicides and attempted suicides in America.*
Young schizophrenics are especially prone to try suicide. Every day in this country more than three hundred people attempt to take their own lives. If the schizophrenic knew that he is the victim of a "metabolic error" in his body, which produces poisonous substances that affect his brain and cause perception disturbances and radical changes in his thoughts, personality, and behavior, he might not become so despondent. And, if he had some assurance that this poison in his body could be overcome so that he might lead a fairly normal life, the suicide rate among schizophrenics would drop to practically nothing.

Several unrelated studies by physicians in the United States and Europe have indicated that some suicides were the result of magnesium deficiency. Experimental studies on animals show that a magnesium deficiency caused the subjects to become hysterical at the sight of shadows and at the sound of small noises. The relationship between magnesium and mental health has not, so far as we are able to determine, been absolutely established, but preliminary studies and tests strongly indicate that magnesium brings mental stability. Perhaps within the next few years it will be definitely established that magnesium is vital to mental health.

We cannot forget that the callous attitude of many psychiatrists toward mental patients, as shown later by letters from patients and their parents, has done nothing to ward off the suicide of young, despondent patients.

9. *Schizophrenia generally strikes persons who have theretofore been relatively normal.*
This is the reason the experience is so terrifying. It interferes with normal communication with others, thus isolating the schizophrenic from his family and friends.

The disease may strike at any age (babies may be born with it), but it takes its greatest toll of those in the 16-to-30 age group. Breakdowns in college (schizophrenia) are not uncommon.

10. *The emotional factors in schizophrenia cannot be discounted.*
Many professionals contend that negative emotions, such as fear and hatred, despair and self-pity, can upset body chemistry and produce toxins that poison the brain.

While love is a powerful therapy in the treatment of any type of mental illness, we now know that love and tender care alone cannot cure a physical disease, whether it be schizophrenia, diabetes, tuberculosis, heart disease, or whatever the disease is.

The A.S.F. has repeatedly warned against self-diagnosis and self-medication. It has, however, in general terms, pointed out some signs of schizophrenia which everyone should know. We shall briefly list the disturbances common to nearly all schizophrenics.

(A) PERCEPTUAL CHANGES IN SEEING, HEARING, TOUCH-ING, TASTING, AND SMELLING. The inner and the outer worlds of a normal person are fairly constant or consistent. If a normal person is given a hallucinatory drug such as LSD, his perceptions are distorted. His normal senses of hearing, feeling, tasting, smelling, and seeing will be so distorted that he may not be able to trust any of these. So it is with the schizophrenic who finds that he cannot rely on his sensory experiences as before. Naturally he panics, fearing that he is losing his mind.

(B) DISTURBANCES IN THOUGHT. The schizophrenic may become the victim of delusions and/or hallucinations. For example, his change in perception of the taste of foods may lead him to believe that his wife is trying to poison him. Other perceptual changes may lead him to believe that a stranger walking behind him has the appearance of a dangerous enemy.

(C) CHANGES IN MOOD. Deep depression, crippling fa-tigue, overwhelming fear, and severe inner tension are characteristic of schizophrenics.

From those who have recovered, we have learned that the inner world of the schizophrenic is turbulent and terrifying, sometimes seeming to be beyond human en-durance. It is no wonder these people sometimes do not know who they are, and often claim to be persons who died years before.

(D) CHANGES IN BEHAVIOR. Because of his changes in perception, thought, and mood, the schizophrenic may have unreasonable changes in behavior. If, without justi-fiable cause, he feels that he is about to be harmed, he may take either defensive or offensive action that might result in the injury or death of another.

Most of the persons arrested in recent years for threatening the lives of American Presidents were schizophrenics. They may have believed that the President was persecuting them.

The purpose of the A.S.F. can be summarized in one short phrase: *to bring about a new dignity for schizophrenics.* As the Fort Worth *Star Telegram* so aptly said of the Foundation, "An organization whose sole and total commitment is to find a cure for the mental plague of the century should receive the moral and financial support it needs for the task."

# 6

# Schizophrenia
# responds favorably
# to vitamin therapy

Scientists have known for some time that when various poisonous substances are extracted from the blood and urine of schizophrenics and injected into the blood of normal persons, such persons will have many of the classic symptoms of schizophrenia.

Psychiatrists are aware that whatever the cause of the toxins in the body of the schizophrenic, they affect his brain and cause him to live in a different world from that of normal individuals. A tremendous amount of scientific evidence has been accumulated showing that the schizophrenic is the victim of some kind of metabolic error in his body chemistry.

Schizophrenics, in or out of hospitals, are generally given no information about their illness, its cause, or its diagnosis. About all loving relatives are told is that the psychiatrists are in hopeless conflict as to the cause of the disease.

According to two eminent psychiatrists, Dr. Abram Hoffer and Dr. Humphry Osmond, "Before anyone can get schizophrenia, his body 'factory' must be different from that of a normal subject in that it must have the capacity to go out of order for some reason and start biochemical changes in motion. That is an essential cause of schizophrenia. Without it, the disease cannot occur. With it, it may occur, but it also may not, just as everyone susceptible to tuberculosis does not develop tuberculosis."

After taking mescaline, a drug derived from a Mexican cactus plant, the late Aldous Huxley commented that "the schizophrenic is like a man permanently under the influence of mescaline."

Professor Mark Altschule, of the Harvard Medical School, and researchers in Paris and Prague have found substances resembling adrenochrome in the urine and blood of schizophrenics.

Dr. Robert Heath, psychiatrist, of Tulane University, has indicated that an abnormal amount of a protein called taraxein is present in the blood of schizophrenics. Less than a millionth of an ounce of taraxein when injected into human volunteers created all the symptoms of schizophrenia.

Using themselves as guinea pigs, Drs. Osmond and Hoffer received intravenous injections of adrenochrome. Ten minutes later, Dr. Osmond noticed that the ceiling had changed color and that the lighting had become brighter. When he left the laboratory, he found that he could not relate distance and time. He found the corridors outside "sinister and unfriendly." Commenting further, he said: "I felt indifferent towards humans and had to curb myself from making unpleasant remarks about them. We had coffee at a wayside halt and here I became disturbed by the covert glances of a sinister-looking man."

Dr. Osmond has been directing mental hospitals in the United States and Canada for over twenty years. Dr. Hoffer is a former director of psychiatric research at the University Hospital in Saskatoon (Canada). Some years ago, Dr. Hoffer lamented, "We badly need new ideas, new methods, new treatments. The older methods aren't doing the job. While schizophrenics fill twenty-five per cent of the world's hospital beds, the recovery rate remains low and the rate of admission high."

The American Schizophrenia Foundation, in its *Newsletter* for October, 1967, reported the recovery or marked improvement of about 80 per cent of schizophrenics treated with vitamin B$_3$ (niacin, or nicotinamide) and vitamin C (ascorbic acid). Twelve psychiatrists, all members of the Foundation's Committee on Therapy, said that large doses of these vitamins, prescribed in combination with other therapies, proved effective with eight out of ten schizophrenia patients. Ten of their papers were published in the *Journal of Schizophrenia* for November 10, 1967 (vol. 1, no. 3).

These twelve physicians worked in widely separated clinics, and, as might be expected, when the patients were found to be hypoglycemic, or suffering from low blood sugar, were given diets to correct such condition.

"This treatment approach is extremely economical and within the reach of every family," observed Dr. David Hawkins, director of the North Nassau Mental Health Center, Manhasset, N.Y. "Of considerable importance for community psychiatry was the discovery that infrequent patients' visits spaced at increasing intervals were quite sufficient for most patients under the vitamin therapy."

Dr. Willard Beebe, a prominent Michigan psychiatrist, said, "For all practical purposes, our committee members have individually confirmed the basic work that was begun in Saskatchewan in the early fifties by Dr. Abram Hoffer and Dr. Humphry Osmond."

Dr. J. Ross MacLean, director of Hollywood Psychiatric Hospital, New Westminister, B.C. (Canada), reported that since 1961 he had treated 350 cases of schizophrenia with vitamins $B_3$ and C, and that even among the chronic, relapsing schizophrenics "there was a substantial improvement in their clinical condition, as evidenced by a reduction in the number of admissions and in the number of days per admission compared to their history of an equivalent period before niacin was started. . . . Patients remain cooperative and hopeful to an extent that I had not seen before in my practice."

Dr. Hawkins reported that fifty-two adult schizophrenics given a minimum daily dose of four grams of vitamin $B_3$ (niacin) and two grams daily of vitamin C (ascorbic acid) recovered, or were greatly improved. "The improvement rate was surprisingly high in view of the fact that 50 per cent of the patients had already had previous treatment elsewhere," commented Dr. Hawkins.

Dr. Jack Ward, noted New Jersey psychiatrist, reported on fifty-nine schizophrenic patients given the vitamin therapy. He found that 86 per cent responded favorably. "Many patients whom I would ordinarily see once weekly for a year or two, I now see for a total of six to ten interviews," said Dr. Ward.

Dr. Allan Cott, a leading New York psychiatrist, reported that fifty of seventy ambulatory schizophrenic patients treated with vitamins were either improved, or much improved. All of the patients had been ill for years and had been previously treated by psychotherapy, electric shock, and hospitalization.

Dr. Joseph Tobin, noted Wisconsin psychiatrist, commented that his clinical experiences confirmed the work of Drs. Osmond and Hoffer, and that a diligent search of medical literature failed to show a single case where negative results were reported with the niacin therapy.

Reliable estimates show that between 1,500 and 2,000 physicians in the United States and more than one hundred institutions are now successfully using the vitamin therapy—more accurately, the megavitamin therapy—with diagnosed schizophrenics and that the cost of the vitamins is less than ten cents a day per patient.

Drs. Osmond and Hoffer readily admit that the new method of treating schizophrenics with vitamins is far from perfect. Dr. Osmond said, "It's still a relatively crude therapy, but a step in the right direction," and Dr. Hoffer commented, "It will probably go through many refinements, and we're all very eager to see something better developed."

In January, 1967, eighty clinical psychiatrists, mostly from the staffs of mental hospitals, met with the originators of the vitamin therapy, Drs. Hoffer and Osmond, to hear discussions of the new technique for treating schizophrenics. These eighty physicians were told by Dr. Hoffer and by Dr. Osmond that they had successfully treated more than five hundred schizophrenics, enabling these patients to return to their homes, to work, and to lead fairly normal lives so long as they continued the vitamin therapy periodically.

Several theories have been advanced as to how the vitamin treatment helps schizophrenics. It seems to be generally agreed that the underlying cause is metabolic inadequacy. Much evidence has been accumulated showing that the schizophrenic is the victim of an inner poisoner, a defect in his body chemistry that causes him to brew, perhaps in his liver, maybe in his adrenal glands, some substance that distorts the working of his brain. This brain poison produces psychological changes in perception, thought, mood, and behavior so that the hallmark of schizophrenia is a change in personality.

It has been suggested that a schizophrenic's body may not be able to produce some enzyme, making it impossible for him to properly utilize vitamin $B_3$ from his food, as does the average individual. Some physicians believe that massive doses of vitamins help to raise the blood sugar level of the hypoglycemic-schizophrenic person, and that this overcomes the toxic bodily condition. Another view is that the vitamins destroy the toxic metabolic products in the blood of schizophrenics.

One cured schizophrenic wrote, "It's really not important to me how or why the vitamin therapy works. All that matters is that after eleven years of a living hell, I am *well!*"

Dr. Roy R. Grinker, Sr., a psychiatrist, writing in a recent issue of the *Journal of the American Medical Association*, said, "Psychiatry and psychoanalysis have not lived up to their well-advertised and hoped-for promise.

One has only to talk to disappointed patients and confused and frustrated therapists to ascertain this." Dr.
Grinker went on to say that what psychiatry desperately
needs is a scientific basis.

Dr. Osmond, in a postscript to *In Search of Sanity* by
Gregory Stefan, observed, "A hundred years ago, Oliver
Wendell Holmes and Ignaz Semmelweis—the pioneer
advocates of antiseptics—urged the medical profession to
take the simple precaution of washing hands before going
from the autopsy table to the delivery room. Today, it
seems beyond belief that their medical colleagues could
have rashly or heedlessly resisted the simple counsel. Yet
Semmelweis and Holmes were not only ignored; they
were persecuted.

"Medical men have their habits and their traditions.
They are creatures of custom much like the rest of us.

"Today, there are still psychiatrists who believe that
grave illnesses such as schizophrenia are caused primarily
by disturbances in social and emotional development—
one of the older, more respectable and less useful medical
ideas which have been applied to a great number of illnesses at one time or another."

According to a recent article in the *British Journal of
Psychiatry*, physicians who go into psychiatry may themselves need psychiatric aid. "Psychiatry as a specialty
may attract more doctors themselves in need of psychiatric help," the report said, after examining the records
of nearly two hundred physicians (mostly psychiatrists)
treated at two British hospitals. Other conclusions in the
report were that doctors' marriages broke down more
readily than others in the same social class; and that drug

addiction was significantly higher and 25 per cent of the doctors discharged themselves from hospitals against advice.

Dr. James Folsom, director of the Veterans Administration Hospital at Tuscaloosa, Ala., recently reported the discovery of a new substance called "friendliness," which, when applied by his hospital staff, yielded notable improvement in the well-being of schizophrenic patients. Dr. Folsom admitted that he braved stiff opposition to such a revolutionary treatment.

Dr. Edwin Dunlop, a Massachusetts psychiatrist, believes that doctors share a large part of the responsibility for suicides in this country. He recently told the Ontario branch of the College of General Practice that 50 per cent of suicides are "the result of neglected medical treatment."

Dr. J. D. W. Pearce, a British psychiatrist, in discussing changes in mental hospitals, said, "In the old days we had the closed door, then the open door, and now we have the revolving door."

Some doctors who are accustomed to prescribing vitamins in minute doses have questioned the advisability of giving schizophrenics massive doses of vitamins. Dr. Hoffer said that niacin ($B_3$) has been used in large doses in heart disease, alcoholism, and arthritis without ill effects. "Niacin," said Dr. Hoffer, "is much less toxic than tranquilizers and antidepressants, and it is probably safer than aspirin."

Dr. Osmond, speaking to more than two hundred persons at a public forum in Ann Arbor, Mich., on May 14, 1967, said that schizophrenia could possibly be eliminated in the next fifteen to twenty years if we work hard enough at it. He pointed out that polio (poliomyelitis) had virtually been eliminated through the giant research effort started by the late President Roosevelt through the March of Dimes. A similar effort, he said, could produce the same results with schizophrenia.

It should be observed that while the American Schizophrenia Foundation is doing an amazing job, considering its available finances, of furnishing physicians and laymen with the latest available information in the search for the best methods of treating schizophrenia, it refuses to approve or endorse any method of treatment discussed.

Schizophrenics Anonymous, a group of people diagnosed as having had schizophrenia, was organized to give its members mutual support and inspiration, and to assist other schizophrenics to recover their mental health. With international headquarters in Canada and local chapters in cities and towns in Canada and the United States, this organization is carrying on a valiant battle to help medical science eradicate schizophrenia. Particularly helpful to nonmembers has been the group's distribution of literature about the disease and its work in supplying names and addresses of psychiatrists who have had success in treating schizophrenia with the vitamin therapy.

Drs. Hoffer and Osmond, in *How to Live with Schizophrenia*, commented, "We consider that helping the patient learn about his disease, and teaching him to become aware of what he can expect because of it, is an important part of treatment. . . . We discuss symptoms frankly. If, for example, you are frightened because objects appear to get larger as they get closer, a well-known but irritating symptom, or if you were to complain about extreme fatigue, we would then explain these as being well-known results of schizophrenia due to disturbances produced in the brain by the illness. If you are suffering from delusions, we would tell you so and explain them as delusions."

To summarize: the megavitamin therapy of treating schizophrenia has nothing to do with vitamin deficiencies or vitamin requirements. Doctors who use the megavitamin therapy know that the mental illness was not caused by vitamin deficiencies. It is true that the patients frequently actually do have vitamin requirements, but the prescribed dosages in such cases are near the ordinary daily requirements.

In the megavitamin therapy, vitamins are not used as vitamins, but as harmless and very useful chemicals intended to balance faulty body chemistry. The vitamins prescribed are inexpensive, can be taken orally, and have no dangerous side effects, even if taken in large amounts over long periods of time. Physicians report that some of their patients have taken massive doses of vitamins for over fifteen years with no adverse effects. Doctors also point out that these vitamins may safely be used in combination with other medication, when required for any kind of physical or mental illness.

Perhaps because of their conservative training, most physicians hesitate to prescribe the larger dosages of vitamins necessary to cure schizophrenia. Sometimes this may be a thousand times the minimum daily requirement set by the vitamin manufacturer. This is why it is called the *megavitamin therapy*. It is also frequently referred to as the *niacin therapy*, which may appear to be misleading, because niacin itself may not always be used—some other form of vitamin B₃ may be prescribed.

Psychiatrists always remind us that the megavitamin therapy is not to be used in the place of other successful and recognized therapies, but always in combination with them. Doctors use tranquilizers, sedatives, antidepressants, other drugs, and shock treatments. They also recommend proper diet, physical exercise, rest, supportive psychotherapy, and group therapy. A spiritual program is also helpful.

No person with mental illness of any kind should start treating himself with massive doses of vitamins. He will need a doctor because generally he should have other medication that only a physician can and may safely prescribe. The megavitamin therapy makes other drugs, when required, more effective. However, doctors usually find that the supporting tranquilizers, sedatives, antidepressants, and other drugs may gradually be reduced and later dispensed with entirely. A good book for physicians is Dr. Abram Hoffer's *Niacin Therapy in Psychiatry* (Charles C Thomas, Publisher, Springfield, Ill., 1962).

Further discussion of the new method of treating schizophrenia will be found in Appendix C.

# 7

# "You will never know the hell I endured"

No physician and no layman can describe the suffering of a schizophrenic quite as vividly as can the patient himself or as can a close relative who has lived with the schizophrenic.

With the help of the American Schizophrenia Foundation and Schizophrenics Anonymous, we have secured many letters from schizophrenics and the immediate members of their families. We quote from some of these:

"My name is Irene. I was released from a large mental hospital in Ontario in 1965. I came to Vancouver to be with my sister and because of my close contact with S.A. [Schizophrenics Anonymous] many necessary 'helps' to aid myself in keeping well. I was in the hospital the last time for ten years and was labeled on my discharge as chronic schizophrenic (unspecified type). I felt as though I was stepping into a strange new world. Everything had changed except me. There was a void in my life, because time ceased to pass by while I was in the hospital.

"I wanted to pick up where I had left off years before. Through the S.A. programme I learned that many schizophrenics go through this experience and must work out new habits and create a whole new outlook on life, one day at a time. This way we create a new presence, a hopeful future, and a dead past. Unpleasant memories are best forgotten and can be if I have a conscious contact with today. I started on vitamin B-3 a year and a half ago, and it has truly given me a kind of life I've never experienced. Until then I was on a medication that did keep my nerves under control but, unfortunately for me, kept me in a state of complete fatigue.

"The B-3 seems to put the vitality in my constitution that I feel the other medication must have stifled. It has helped me to concentrate and think clearly. Because of this, I started to get my self-confidence back and then I started 'feeling' things again. Like my emotions began to work again. I started to feel friendly with people. I was able to share an experience and relate to people and really started to live again.

"The first year and a half that I was out of the hospital I lived with my sister. The last year and a half I live in my own little two-room suite, and manage my own affairs. I know I must follow the aids that have been proven to keep people like me well. I used to hate taking pills, until I learned *why* I had to take them and now it is not too bad. I feel very grateful because I meet others at the Group who are not as well as I. Many of my friends back at the hospital may never be as lucky as I was and I know this. If there was more understanding and information given to the families of schizophrenics, so many of these people could be given the chance of living again.

Irene
British Columbia"

"About fifteen years ago I started suffering from a general rundown condition and extreme depression. The rundown condition was easy enough to remedy; however, I was still not able to alleviate the depression in any way. I saw a psychiatrist for this condition and I began extensive therapy. . . . My depression did not change, and at this point I hied myself off to an internist who willingly gave me some amphetamine (small doses) to lift my moods. I would like to add here that I had low blood pressure, a low metabolic rate, and a general sluggish condition, and I did take iron pills and other vitamins for this, but still the depression did not lift and it was as a result of this that the internist prescribed the amphetamine.

"Needless to say that I felt greatly improved, and of course although I ate well I did not feel the need for special dietary control. It wasn't too long before I became hallucinatory and had to be admitted to a mental hospital. This was under the care of the psychiatrist, and true to his nature, I was labeled 'schizophrenic.' After a few shock treatments and withdrawal of the amphetamine, I returned to normal, but I and my parents were told that I was an extremely mentally ill person and perhaps even incurable.

"I was discharged, therapy was continued even more extensively, and greater personality changes took place— but not the depression. (At this point, of course, I believed I was mentally ill.) So, again I got my hands on some amphetamine (this time from the psychiatrist) and the same thing occurred again.

"Believe it or not, this same circle of events continued

for the next ten years, with my being hospitalized about once each year as a result of what I later learned was 'sugar starvation' of the brain.

"Thinking I was schizophrenic . . . I learned of Dr. Hoffer's work in Canada and the niacinamide. This did not particularly apply to me; however, in his work he mentioned that a lot of patients were hypoglycemic (low blood sugar) and that this condition causes depression. I had a blood sugar test run and indeed I was hypoglycemic, and quite critically.

"I treated this condition with drastic diet for three months, followed by a modified diet, also took thyroid pills occasionally to help that condition and some iron, and my depression lifted within a week's time. I continue to treat my hypoglycemia with a modified diet and common sense and I at last feel more pep and certainly no depression of the order I had known. This, of course, means that I have no need for any amphetamines and I have not been sick since. (The danger with amphetamines, especially to those who actually need them, is that one will stop eating so that the sugar supply to the brain is cut off and this is what causes the hallucinations. Most people who actually crave this drug are hypoglycemics, so that this circle of events is easily produced.)

"My biggest problem is simply maintaining the will power to handle my hypoglycemic condition by diet. And, believe me, just knowing what the problem is has been a blessing. . . . Because of improper diet I became a 'mental case.' The whole thing is like a bad dream now and I would prefer not to have been born than to have to go through with that again.

"When I think of the money we have spent and the things we have listened to from all those psychiatrists, I can hardly believe it to be true. Sometimes when I am alone I ask myself, 'How could this have happened to me?'

D. J. B.
Washington, D.C."


"I have seemingly recovered from a chronic condition of schizophrenia through biochemical and physical treatment after seeking help for sixteen years with every other known treatment.

"Research in the past decade has led many researchers to believe that a defect in body chemistry causes a victim of schizophrenia to brew a poison in his system due to a malfunction of the adrenal glands or perhaps the liver. Dr. Abram Hoffer of Canada and Dr. Humphry Osmond of New Jersey developed a megavitamin treatment to 'mop' up this poison which causes distortion of the senses, thought, and mood. This theory proved valid in my case. I have been on the megavitamin treatment for two years. I take 3,000 mg. of niacin and 3,000 mg. of vitamin C daily. Along with this I take vitamin B-1, B-2, B-6, and B-12 and vitamin E in very large amounts, plus an all-vitamin with minerals.

"I am also on a hypoglycemia diet for low blood sugar. Though I am on the above treatment and am well, in the past I have had tranquilizers, antidepressants, sleeping medication, hormones, and a series of electroshock therapy. . . .

"Through the program and steps of Schizophrenics Anonymous I have developed a positive and spiritual outlook on life. I have learned to live within limitations, reserving my energy and, above all, getting sufficient rest along with adequate exercise. All factors have contributed to my recovery.

"The medical treatment is specialized—few doctors in California know about it and few believe in it, though I know from experience it is valid. However, I doubt the medical treatment would suffice for total recovery without the change to spiritual values and change in living style.

"The massive dose of vitamins seems to do a fine job of 'mopping' the toxins out of the system, but is no value without applying the common sense health rules for schizophrenics. Primarily, the vitamins acted as a tool. With a lessening of the toxin, I was able to help myself. Knowledge about the disease and association with other schizophrenics were very helpful.

"Because research in schizophrenia is going on now at a more rapid pace on the body chemistry theory, I would not in my own mind rule out nutrition as a contributing factor. However, it seems to be a complex problem with many factors at this time. I do believe nutrition is a very important part of mental health and believe we are semi-starved with modern packaging methods and a diet too rich in sugar and starch. Also, I wonder how all the modern drugs affect our body chemistry.

"If I can be of any further help, please let me know.

MARGARET D.
California"

"Fortunately, I came in contact with Schizophrenics Anonymous a few months ago.

"Presently I am taking four grams of niacin in the course of a day and I am getting results; symptoms that have been with me for about thirty years have left me.

"Recently at a meeting of Schizophrenics Anonymous I was told that it is sometimes necessary to give schizophrenics 25 grams of niacin a day to get best results. For me a mere 150 mg. of niacin a day did no good.

"In addition to the niacin I also take three grams of vitamin C a day, as advised. The proper hygiene we follow also includes eating a high-protein diet with no sweets, no coffee, plus enough sleep and exercise every day. We may not yet know all about the disease, but we know it has a chemical-physical basis and are now on the right track. Surely millions of people have this disease and don't know it.

M. P.
New York"


"I am available at all times to help the Schizophrenic Foundation when needed, as the niacin therapy has cured my 'emotional disease,' my arthritis, and has given me many other benefits. Lately, however, I have confined my efforts to the alcoholics with severe emotional problems, depressions, fatigue, etc. At my suggestion, forty or fifty people have started the B-3 vitamin therapy and all of them are getting tremendous results! If you would like to have case histories of those who have gotten such wonderful help from niacin (including my own story) I will gladly get them for you.

VIRGINIA
California"


"I am a member of a group called 'Parents of Hippies,' meeting in the Washington, D.C., area. Besides providing mutual sympathy for our various heartaches, we have been investigating many different aspects of this phenomena among our young people. Our collective experience with psychologists, psychiatrists and sociologists is great. We have heard ourselves and society blamed.

"Lately, we have had representatives of local chapters of Health Frontiers (hypoglycemia) and the American Schizophrenic Foundation meet with us.

"The idea that our children's apathy, withdrawal, antisocial behavior, and drug involvement may have a *physiological* explanation is both enlightening and encouraging. In comparing notes with other parents, it would seem that a high percentage of our 'hippie' children suffer from nutritional deficiencies—as compared with our own 'nonhippie' children.

ELIZABETH
Maryland"


"I have learned from practical experience, having been a psychiatric patient suffering from schizophrenia for the past five years, that proper nutrition is fundamental to mental health.

"In the last eight months I have been on a high-protein, low-carbohydrate diet and the change has been amazing. My energy has increased, and I have found that eating or drinking high-protein foods often during the day enables me to avoid fatigue and that common hell known as depression, which often accompanies it.

"As a schizophrenic, I have also learned that avoiding certain foods is necessary—namely, cheese (except cottage cheese and cream), caffeine and cigarettes. These all contain taraxacin which is toxic to the schizophrenic. Another thing of interest is that over fifty per cent of schizophrenics suffer from hypoglycemia, or low blood sugar. It is extremely important that these people avoid anything with a high content of sugar, as well as the things named above (cheese, caffeine, and cigarettes). It is also important that these people eat often, or their blood sugar level will drop and they will experience uncomfortable psychological symptoms, such as depression or lightness of the head.

"I will now attempt to give a fairly complete list of the things which a person with hypoglycemia should avoid: cheese, anything made with sugar, potatoes, rice, cereals, spaghetti, macaroni, noodles, wines, cordials, cocktails, and beer.

"In the past it was not realized that biochemistry and nutrition play a part in mental illness, but today, through this realization, we are able to help ourselves by following a proper diet (and through the use of such drugs and vitamins as are prescribed). Here I am referring to the megavitamin therapy now being used to treat schizophrenia, which has enabled me to re-enter the world as it truly is.

DONALD J. F.
New York"


A young woman, apparently highly intelligent, wrote that, although she had been in and out of mental hospitals several times, had received repeated shock treatments, and had nothing to look forward to except incarceration, she now finds life exciting and worthwhile. Her letter continues:

"I found out from Dr. _____ that it is possible I may never have to be hospitalized for schizophrenia again! I don't know if you can imagine how much this means to me. It's like someone handing my life back to me. Schizophrenia is brought on by a chemical imbalance produced by caffeine and carbohydrates, which some individuals cannot assimilate. This produces toxins which affect the brain and the senses of taste, sight, and smell. I am on a lifetime diet now of high-protein foods and absolutely no caffeine or carbohydrates! With the diet and 3,000 milligrams of nicotinamide per day, I can maintain my system's chemical balance for the rest of my life. For that I am very grateful!

B.D.
Washington"

"I'm proud of my charter membership card in the American Schizophrenia Foundation and it is being placed in a frame with other treasures as a constant reminder of its meaning. I deplore the anonymity tagged on the organizations to help those of us with mental and emotional problems, and I look forward to the day when we need be no more ashamed of our illness than a person with any one of dozens of ailments that can be named.

K. S.
Illinois"

The following letter was written to a member of Schizophrenics Anonymous:

"Your organization and American Schizophrenia Foundation saved my life, my marriage, and have given me reason to be optimistic about the future. For the first time in more than a year, I *feel* happy and look forward to each new day. . . . Words are inadequate to thank you, but that is all we have.

E. A.
Oregon"

"Our son's improvement has been tremendous. We're almost afraid to believe it. . . . The Osmond-Hoffer book [*How to Live With Schizophrenia*] should be required reading for all doctors. . . .

R. J.
New Hampshire"

"Even though the niacin therapy got me over the terrible depression, fatigue and exhaustion I had while in the mental hospital, it was Schizophrenics Anonymous that got me to where I could enjoy life again.

"It was a long time after I left the hospital before I could do these things:

"Start doing the dishes or a washing without being afraid I would start breaking the dishes or tearing the clothes.

"Walk down the street without feeling that every person I met wanted to hurt me.

"Get in a bus without being afraid that everyone was laughing at me.

"Turn on the radio without being afraid of hearing voices telling me to kill myself.

"Eat food I had not seen prepared without fearing that I would be poisoned.

"Enjoy bright colors again after years of the gray world of schizophrenia.

"We schizophrenics want to get well. We do not enjoy our world of perceptual distortions. We want more than anything else to get back to meaningful and productive living.

"Most doctors and many psychiatrists just don't understand how destructive schizophrenia is. It destroys financially and socially. It destroys the entire human being. It destroys the family.

O. D.
Saskatchewan, Canada."

"Only those who have experienced it know the strain which one sick member can have on the whole family, and the wonderful relief when the child is well.

"Our daughter is now back in school in the grade she would normally have been in had she never been ill, and she is getting good marks.

"The psychiatrist, after prolonged treatment, said she had permanent brain damage. He recommended, for the sake of the family, that this 'hopelessly' sick child be put in an institution. I was never able to believe his diagnosis since at intervals she had been normal and bright. I could not understand how this could be if the brain had been 'permanently impaired.'

"We found another specialist who recommended the megavitamin therapy. Thank God, it worked, and she is well now!

"I think Schizophrenics Anonymous should concentrate on the education of the families of schizophrenics since their understanding of the patient's problems is so important for a return to health of the sick member for the preservation of a good family life.

M. O.
New York"

Gregory Stefan, in his book *In Search of Sanity*, re-calls the greatest tragedy of his life—when his wife, still very much in love with him, obtained a divorce while he was in a mental hospital because a psychiatrist had talked her into believing that a divorce was the best way to help her husband recover. He also relates the terrible ordeals of other mental patients in the same hospital who had their marriages destroyed by divorces obtained by spouses outside the hospital at the insistence of psychiatrists.

"When my husband and I were asked to give a home to a small schizophrenic boy, we were undecided. We finally agreed to talk with the mother of the child.

"The next day Mrs. B. (the boy's mother) and a friend of hers brought Tommy over to meet us. One look at his unhappy face and his mother's pleading one made us decide to at least give him a temporary home.

"Tommy was an undersized, forlorn looking child. His clothes hung limply on his skinny frame and his hair was either shaved off or clipped very short. He had a peculiar twitch to his face and he sort of dragged his feet when he walked, making shuffling noises.

"He did not talk at all that evening except to answer the few questions that were asked of him. Then he'd barely raise his voice above a whisper. Later on, to our despair, we discovered he could certainly use that voice when he'd fly into one of his rages.

"We gave him one of our two bedrooms downstairs. The other one is occupied by our son. I was amazed to see boxes in his room which I thought contained his clothes. These boxes contained Mad Magazines, comics and horror books.

"In the beginning, Tommy stayed in his room most of the time. We left him alone. Then, slowly, he started mingling with the family. One day he asked me if he could hang a few pictures on the wall of his room, to which I agreed. When I went down to see what he was doing, I was quite unprepared for what I saw. All of the walls were *pasted* with pictures cut out of Mad Magazines and jokes. When I asked him to stop damaging the walls, he flew into a rage and we had quite a time calming him down.

"Tommy used to put me through all sorts of tests, such as rattling a dish, or making unnecessary noises while staring straight at me. I would try to ignore this, but he would not stop when I asked him to do so. He would continue on and on until, in exasperation, I'd give him a spanking, after which he would run down to his room and sulk for hours.

"Tommy suffered from delusions of grandeur. He imagined he was far superior in intelligence to other children. He *was* intelligent and interested in science. If you agreed with him, he would keep on talking about outer-space flying and the supernatural. If one disagreed with him, he became furious.

"Tommy was very moody. One minute he'd be very happy (high) and acting up. The next, he would be bitter, argumentative and depressed. He complained of headaches and blurry vision, but the eye specialist found nothing wrong with his eyes.

"He told us he hated his mother and refused to write or 'phone her. We tried to encourage him to like his mother and explained that she had not had him committed to an institution because she loved him and was afraid of losing him.

"Dr. _____ recommended massive doses of vitamin B₃ (nicotinamide). To get him to take these pills was an ordeal. He would toss the pills up in the air or roll them around on the table until they were broken into pieces. He liked pizzas, and I finally prevailed on him to take the vitamin pills by making pizzas for him.

"Tommy improved slowly. He got to where he was taking his pills regularly without any fuss. We noticed that he idolized our seventeen-year-old son. He became friendly and full of fun. He learned to be considerate of others. One morning I was sick and unable to get up. When Tommy came to my door and knocked, I asked him to get his own breakfast. He offered to get something for me, which pleased me very much. His attitude toward his mother changed and he wrote and 'phoned her regularly. Thanks to nicotinamide, Tommy became a wonderful boy.

Mrs. N.
Saskatchewan, Canada"

"Our baby cried a lot, but otherwise seemed normal enough. She displayed early talents in speech and singing. At eighteen months of age, she was singing herself to sleep every night. By two years she had quite a 'repertoire' of nursery rhymes and folk songs.

"At the age of three she began to have depressions out of all proportion to reason. She would sit for hours in these moods, or would eat things like worms from the garden, or would run away without clothing.

"Our little girl was always tired and exhausted. I am

a teacher and my husband has a business so she spent much time with her grandmother. Even though my mother was kind to her, she considered our little girl a nuisance because her behavior was 'different.' Her grandmother called her a 'bold, bad girl,' which wasn't true.

"One person understood the child and loved her. She was her aunt who was schizophrenic. The child could relate with dear Aunt Ida. There seemed to be a fond rapport between them. The aunt was childless and had doted on her niece since birth. The easy-going pace of the one calmed the other.

"Then came school. She suffered anemia, vertigo, nausea, eye reversal, blurring and many other symptoms. The doctor said she was a paranoid and should be put in an institution. However, we did not agree with the doctor.

"One grade seemed like another. There was a fog of mind that did not lift until she was in grade nine. Her marks rose all year until she was seventh from the top of her class. She felt now that high school would be clear sailing. She loved her books and worked hard. We had moved to a larger house so she had the advantage of having a room of her own. This year of happiness was the last she was to know for years.

"The next few years were all pretty much alike, failure in school, visual hallucinations, depression and exhaustion. We had heard of Dr. Hoffer's success in treating schizophrenia with vitamin therapy. Our physician contacted Dr. Hoffer and found out how much vitamin $B_3$ to give our daughter.

"With this treatment she became a different person. The mental fog lifted, the depression and fatigue vanished and life was good for her. At nineteen our daughter began a new, exciting and thrilling life. It all seems like a wonderful dream to us, but we know it is real.

"So much heartache and suffering for our little girl could have been avoided if doctors had known about the vitamin therapy when she first showed schizophrenic symptoms.

Mrs. S. P.
Alberta, Canada"

"I am a new, but happy member of Schizophrenics Anonymous. These are some of the things I learned to do at my first meetings:

"1.   Eat a balanced and nutritious diet.

"2.   Follow a daily program of physical exercise.

"3.   Take some time out each day for sport or other recreation.

"4.   Live within my reserves.

"5.   Take a tepid bath daily—the cheapest and best tranquilizer.

"6.   Get sufficient sleep every night. Most schizophrenics suffer from fatigue and lack of energy, consequently we need more sleep and rest than do other persons.

"7.   Avoid all drugs, particularly tranquilizers, unless prescribed by a qualified physician.

M. D.
Illinois"

"When I was a senior in college I had what the doctors called a 'nervous breakdown.' This was followed by years of treatment by psychiatrists and eventual incarceration in a mental hospital.

"After my release from the hospital a friend gave me *Goodbye Allergies*, a book on hypoglycemia. I found myself on about every page of this book. My local physician was amused when I told him I thought my 'mental illness' resulted from starvation of my brain due to insufficient blood sugar. He said, 'How can a layman know anything about hypoglycemia?' The doctor assured me that the high-protein, low-carbohydrate and medium-fat diet would do no good but was harmless. He warned me that there were hundreds of diet fad books on the market.

"The Seale Harris-Tintera diet and vitamin supplements were all I needed to regain my health, physically and mentally. For more than a year I have been reading books on psychiatry. I am convinced that Sigmund Freud, the idol of those psychiatrists who took so much money from my parents and gave nothing in return, was a fake and a fraud. I was reared in a religious home, and when I read that Freud referred to religion as an 'illusion' and something men would eventually outgrow, I became more disgusted than ever with physicians who have been fooled by the atheistic teachings of this man.

C. F.
California"


"Last August I had a sudden attack of acute schizophrenia and was hospitalized three months.

"When I left the hospital three months later, I was thirty pounds overweight, rundown, depressed, and fearful.

"Since I had received no help or advice, I decided to do so on my own research and while so doing encountered *How to Live With Schizophrenia* by Abram Hoffer and Humphry Osmond, which told of the B-3 treatment for schizophrenics.

"Within an hour after taking massive doses of niacinide my depression vanished, not to return. In a month I had a complete personality change. Self-confidence returned, fear left. I became vibrant, alert, energetic. Friends were amazed.

JOHN A. S.
California"

The following is a copy of a letter sent the author by a member of Schizophrenics Anonymous, who vouched for its authenticity:

"Our daughter's illness was rapidly coming to a climax when she slashed her wrists, which landed her in the psychiatric ward of one of our hospitals. She was delirious and escaped from the ward, climbed out an open window, and jumped seventy-two feet to the ground. When found, she was in a coma and for the next two months she had continuous hallucinations. I was told she would have to be sent to a state hospital and that she was incurably insane.

"I had read in a national magazine of the wonderful work of Dr. Hoffer, and I found a local psychiatrist who was willing to try Dr. Hoffer's method, but who expressed doubt that it would help.

"After a month on niacin, ascorbic acid, other vitamins, and minerals, my daughter appeared to have made remarkable progress. Then she had a relapse. The psychiatrist had only been giving her the dosage for acute cases, so, at my insistence, he prescribed the double dosage needed for chronic cases.

"After nine months, she is a different person! She is in excellent health, pink cheeks, clear skin, firm face, and bright eyes. Before she was hospitalized, she was always tired and despondent, pale, with skin rashes. Her medication is not to be changed for five years.

S.
New York"

"I'll get right to the point. First, I suffer from alcoholism and schizophrenia. I know for sure that I would *not* have stayed sober these five years without the daily use of niacin. I currently take 16 grams a day, along with about 9 grains of ascorbic acid, 16 tablets (200 International Unit size) of vitamin E. I have found amazing results. My thinking is clearer than ever. I do not suffer from fatigue as I used to. I work better because I feel better. I started the vitamin therapy two years ago. I do not think of the time I will need them—that is, I plan to stay on them for the rest of my life.

J. D.
New York"

An active member of Schizophrenics Anonymous wrote that she thought the most inspiring proof of the effectiveness of the megavitamin therapy could be found in the recoveries from mental illness of the members of her group. Her letter continued:

"Dr. ———, a noted child psychiatrist in Vancouver, phoned me to inquire about the S.A. group last week. I mentioned to him the vitamin B-3 that a few of us in our S.A. group are taking, *and* I asked him if he used it. His answer, 'Oh, yes, I've given up to 500 grams a day and it does seem to *perk* up my patients *quite a bit.*' I explained about Dr. A. Hoffer's treatment starting with 3,000 grams up to as high as 10,000 grams to arrest the illness. I have sent this psychiatrist some literature. Unfortunately, here as elsewhere schizophrenia is still considered *and* treated as a psychological illness *only*. I also found out (quite by chance) that our largest mental hospital (Riverview) is now dabbling with using 300 or up to 500 milligrams of vitamin B-3, which does *nothing* to arrest schizophrenia, according to Dr. A. Hoffer. These professional people are the first to sneer and declaim Dr. Hoffer's theory as false. The truth is, as I've found out, that in Vancouver they haven't given anyone near the prescribed dosage, or even bothered to obtain it, which may be obtained free by writing Dr. A. Hoffer. . . . Those who are taking adequate amounts of vitamin B-3 are really different persons in all respects than they were when they started the treatments.

MARGARET
British Columbia"

A member of Schizophrenics Anonymous, who is professor of philosophical psychology in one of our large eastern universities, has prepared an excellent paper for new members of Schizophrenics Anonymous, which we are permitted to use:

### "SCHIZOPHRENIA IS A DISEASE

"When you have schizophrenia you are physically ill. The disease manifests itself in both physical and mental symptoms involving a physical effect on the human brain. Many of the characteristics, such as crippling, fatigue, feelings of listlessness and depression, have a physical base. Even the color of the skin changes to a darker hue and the muscles become flaccid and the eyes manifest a glazed, unnatural look.

"Consequently, the changes which occur affect the responses of the sense organs; the eyes, ears, smelling process, taste, and touch, and also the emotional responses and the actions. Trouble is also obvious in the judgment of time and distance. In the more serious cases there are sight and hearing hallucinations. The very sick schizophrenic actually sees people who do not exist or sees familiar people in a manner in which they do not really exist. Some schizophrenics feel that others are plotting against them and they take measures to protect themselves. Others are quite grandiose and feel that they are in positions of authority or extraordinary success. Others are so rigid that they believe that they will shatter themselves if they move and are frequently found in the one position for long periods of time.

"Schizophrenia is not only a torturous disease involving

severe pain, but it is also a highly complicated disease which involves every single facet of the human personality. Fifty per cent of the patients in mental hospitals are suffering from this disease.

"Sigmund Freud suggested in his writing that the answer to schizophrenia, whether paranoid or catatonic, would very likely be found by the biochemist. Freud thought that many other emotional disturbances were rooted in a biochemical imbalance. This seems to make a great deal of sense because, although the human person is made up of human components, he is still very much a unity. This integration is obvious from the observation of his physical and emotional reactions. These reactions indicate very strongly an interdependence. The physical in part determines the emotional reaction, and the emotional reaction determines in part the quality of the physical response.

"Abram Hoffer, M.D., Ph.D., and Humphry Osmond, M.R.C.S., D.P.M., completely involved themselves in scientific research to find a physical basis for this disease, because most of the schizophrenics whom they had treated over the years through psychotherapy did not get well or stay well. Both of these doctors are highly qualified psychiatrists, biochemists, and medical doctors. Schizophrenia, they thought, was due to a physical change of adrenalin to adrenochrome, which is a toxic poison and an hallucinogen. The toxic poison, according to their theory, passes through the bloodstream, up into the brain cells and affects the transfer of the psychic and physical stimuli which pass from one brain cell to another.

"Actually, the adrenochrome which takes its position

in the synapse, that is, the passageway from one brain cell to another, distorts the perceptual images which were originally received through the healthy sense organs. In other words, the stimuli started out all right, but they ended up distorted because of the adrenochrome.

"These distortions—and there may be many going on at the same time—are the feedback which the human person finds difficult to accept in the first instance. After awhile the distortion is so often repeated, the schizophrenic comes to believe this is the real world and suspects others who do not understand what is going on.

"To base the recovery of the schizophrenic solely on psychotherapy seems to cause the schizophrenic to become more ill. This type of approach is based on the assumption the schizophrenic is not physically ill, that schizophrenia is not a physical disease. When the therapist assumes this, he is basing the process of getting well on something which he has to deny exists at all. Now, if we base our approach to the schizophrenic on the grounds that he is not only mentally unwell, but that he is physically ill, we will be treating the whole person as we find him.

"In an article of this type, it is not possible to treat all the physical and psychological aspects of schizophrenia. Therefore, we will not attempt to do so. The hypothesis which led to finding the biological cause of the disease also led to the solution.

"Drs. Hoffer and Osmond, in the University Hospital of Saskatoon, Canada, over a period of extended research, came to the conclusion that the body of the schizophrenic lacks co-enzyme #1, or NAD. To counteract this genetic deficiency they found that niacin (vitamin B-3), in daily massive doses, interacting with the liver and gastric juices of the stomach, could create enough NAD in most schizophrenics to correct the change of adrenalin into adrenochrome.

"When this capacity to produce NAD out of niacin was not present, both of these doctors were able to correct the deficiency through the intake of pure NAD manufactured from yeast or soybeans. Over a period of 14 years these doctors have treated, along with other doctors who were interested in the megavitamin B-3 therapy, thousands of patients who were readmitted to hospitals many times without success.

"These patients had been treated by other doctors exclusively by extensive psychotherapy to no avail, causing a great deal of frustration in the family of the schizophrenic at an enormous financial outlay. Most of these patients recovered permanently through the use of massive doses of vitamin B-3.

"The question came up as to what kind of psychotherapy should go along with this physical therapy, because after the schizophrenic had suffered many years from emotional distortion, he needed some kind of psychotherapeutic help.

"The experience of Hoffer and Osmond, though somewhat limited, has indicated that group therapy in Schizophrenics Anonymous, like Alcoholics Anonymous for the alcoholic, has proved sufficient. In S.A. the patient follows the same program as the 12 steps of the A.A. program and learns to live out his experience in life through the process of sharing.

"Like the alcoholic, the schizophrenic must face up to the irrevocable fact of the disease even though he is on his way to a cure, and he has to accept the fact that his life became disordered because of the physical and mental components of the disease. He also comes to realize that goal-directed action achieved through shared experience will lead him to a purposeful life. The process of communication which is available to the sick person in S.A. will enable him to communicate adequately with others and with God. In this program he learns how to take care of his body by proper diet, exercise, and rest.

"He learns also in the program he should relate to a competent doctor who is familiar with this therapy. He learns also that he must accept himself as he is, clean up his past, make amends to those whom he has harmed, and re-establish in his life a pattern of spiritual values, and above all bring this message of recovery to other schizophrenics.

"An auxiliary help to the doctor and the patient has been established: The American Schizophrenia Foundation, which has its offices at 305 South State Street, Ann Arbor, Michigan, 48108. This foundation has been established for two reasons: to further continued scientific investigation into the facets of this disease, and to educate society about the disease.

"Hoffer and Osmond have constructed a very useful test which is easy to take and very easy to administer, called the H.O.D. Test. Another test has been fashioned through the research of Hoffer and Abdul El-Meligi, the Experiential World Inventory (EWI), which is available at the Bureau of Research in Neurology and Psychiatry, Neuro-Psychiatric Institute, Princeton, New Jersey.

"The H.O.D. Test is very valid despite its brevity. The EWI indicates in more detail the perceptual distortion and the emotional aberration of the patient. To determine whether or not a patient is schizophrenic, the H.O.D. Test is sufficient. However, if the therapist is anxious to know more about the various facets of the schizophrenic personality, it is also recommended he administer EWI.

"Psychiatrists who are familiar with this disease and with the vitamin B-3 therapy find that they may have to administer *small* doses of tranquilizers, properly chosen and closely regulated. This treatment is also recommended for alcoholics—33 per cent of whom are schizophrenic, according to statistics.

"Hoffer and Osmond have found the megavitamin B-3 therapy is also useful for depressives, those who suffer from neurotic anxiety states, arthritis, and cardiovascular disease.

J. J. R.
New York"

# 8

# Health bonuses galore

When one finds that he should go on a special diet, he is inclined to wonder if the benefits outweigh the annoyance, inconvenience, and other difficulties that go with the diet. The author, from his own experience, hastens to assure the reader that following the hypoglycemia diet is a most pleasant and rewarding way of eating. Space does not permit us to enumerate all of the health benefits, physical and mental, that go with low-carbohydrate, high-protein, and medium-fat nutrition; however, we will discuss a few of them:

1. *Sugar is a contributory cause of heart trouble.*
In three reports appearing in *The Lancet* in 1964, sugar was indicated as one of the causes of heart disease. Dr. John Yudkin, of the University of London, a dietetic specialist, stated that since people who eat fats nearly always eat more sugar, he did not believe that animal fat alone was responsible for heart disease. He cited figures to prove that patients with myocardial infarction consumed more sugar than did normal persons.

Dr. K. J. Kingsbury, according to an article in *The Lancet* for December 24, 1966, reported on 338 male, atherosclerotic patients, chosen at random from mixed social, economic, and occupational classes. This study was

§125

really a continuation of the one done earlier by Dr. Yudkin.

Dr. Kingsbury found that the major cause of heart disease is not fat, but sugar. He showed that an increase in sugar consumption always parallels an increase in heart attacks.

Many scientists, both American and European, have shown how sugar depletes the B vitamins in the body. Two prominent nutritionists, Walter H. Eddy, Ph.D., and Gilbert Dalldorf, M.D., several years ago asserted, "Thiamine deficiency impairs the function of the heart, increases the tendency to extravascular fluid collections, and results in terminal cardiac standstill."

Dr. M. O. Bruker, chief of staff of the Eben-Ezer Hospital (Germany), wrote in an article entitled "Sugar as a Pathogenic" (1962): "Sugar produces relative hypovitaminosis." He then pointed out that in a two-year period in Germany when there was a tremendous increase in sugar consumption, the number of deaths from heart and circulatory diseases rose from 80,000 to 183,000. Dr. Bruker urged everyone who eats sugar (or sugar products) to take more B vitamins, for, as he said, "sugar demands an increased addition of these vitamins."

2. *Chronic fatigue will disappear.*

Dr. Sam E. Roberts, in his recent book *Exhaustion— Causes and Treatment*, asserted that during the last quarter of a century nearly all of the patients who came to him complaining of fatigue or utter exhaustion were suffering from hypoglycemia. Many of them, Dr. Roberts said, had gone through the larger clinics in this country where no successful diagnoses of what caused their perpetual tiredness were made.

3. *Most allergic symptoms will be alleviated.*
These are asthma, hay fever, eczema, hives, food sensitivity, and the like. An adequate discussion of how and why most allergies leave when one is on the antihypoglycemia diet would be too extended for this discussion. The adrenal and pancreatic glands are involved, but, most of all, the cure of nervousness, tension, fatigue, emotional upsets, and resulting general exhaustion, is also a cure for our allergies.

4. *One will age rather slowly.*
This will manifest itself in both the health and in the appearance of the individual on the low-carbohydrate, high-protein, and medium-fat diet. Dr. John W. Tintera and other specialists have found that the tissues of individuals on this diet do not age as rapidly as do the tissues of other persons. Dr. Rudolph Baer and Dr. Sheldon Brodie, both of New York University, writing in the May, 1958, issue of *The Practitioner*, said that adequate nutrition is essential for the preservation of a healthy skin—just as it is for a healthy body. "So it is not surprising that the skin is one of the first and major sites in which vitamin deficiencies manifest themselves," said these doctors, who went on to discuss the separate effects on the skin of vitamins A, B, and C deficiencies.

5. *Eye health is improved.*
Dr. Peter Adams and others, in the July 29, 1967, issue of *The Lancet*, show how vitamin B deficiency impairs

vision. Much medical evidence has been accumulated indicating that a deficiency of riboflavin (vitamin B₂) results in itching and burning of the eyes and bloodshot eyes.

Dr. Donald McLaren, in his book *Malnutrition and the Eye*, traces the experiments made on laboratory rats over a long period to show that these animals when deprived of riboflavin quickly develop eye cataract. Dr. McLaren's book indicates that vitamin E deficiency may have serious effect on the eyes, including possible cataract.

In his book *Deficiency Diseases*, Richard Follis states: "Cataract may develop during the course of deficiencies of protein or of certain vitamins. The lens is likewise affected by amino acid deprivation, though to varying degrees."

Dr. Donald Atkinson presented proof in the February, 1952, *Eye, Ear, Nose and Throat Monthly* that diets rich in vitamins, especially vitamin C, prevented the development of cataracts. "So far as I know," said Dr. Atkinson, "I was the first to prescribe a diet of green tops of garden vegetables to cataract patients."

Several doctors have written that calcium deficiency, or inability to absorb calcium, may be another cause of cataract.

Nearly everyone now knows that a deficiency of vitamin A causes night blindness. Doctors have found that vitamins C and D play an important part in keeping good eyesight.

Since defective eyesight is one of the first indications of old age, and most oldsters have inadequate nutrition, it is imperative that we have good food, with an adequate supply of vitamins and minerals, every day of our lives.

6.  *The mind will never grow old.*

Dr. Irving Lorge, brilliant Columbia University psychologist, has demonstrated that whatever strength of mind one has at twenty or twenty-five he can have at seventy-five, eighty-five, or ninety-five. After explaining the tests he gave to prove that the mind never grows old, Dr. Lorge said, "I believe I am justified in saying that the common belief in the mental decline of older people appears, from these experiments, to be an unfortunate libel. They do not decline mentally at all. The only decline is in speed of reaction. Every older person, indeed anyone beyond forty, is reluctant to concede that he has lost real mental ability. This research indicates that he does not have to concede it. As far as mental ability is concerned, there is no such thing as a 'retiring age.' Men and women both possess the same mental powers in their mature or even advanced years as they had in young manhood and young womanhood."

Dr. Edward L. Thorndike, psychologist, Teachers College, Columbia University, and his associates, aided by a generous grant from The Carnegie Corporation, made studies of the learning abilities of young and older people. The results of these experiments are shown in Professor Thorndike's book *Adult Learning*. After referring to the commonly accepted belief that youngsters learn more easily than do older students, the late Dr. Albert Edward Wiggam said, in *New Techniques of Happiness*, "Professor Thorndike's experiments knock all these notions into a cocked hat."

Calvin P. Stone, of Stanford University, experimented with rats of all ages to determine if there was any difference in the learning abilities of the rat due to age. His conclusion was that the old rats became better in all-around proficiency than the young ones.

Dr. Charles W. Dorland, Chicago physician, studied the lives of four hundred of the world's greatest men and women, and found that many of them had done their greatest work at seventy, and some even at eighty years of age.

Dr. Henry Sherman, famous Columbia University nutrition chemist, caused rats to live one third longer by giving them a special kind of diet, "high protein, high calcium, and high vitamins." More important than merely prolonging life was Dr. Sherman's conclusion that his diet gave the rats a "longer period of buoyant health during old age."

Dr. Robert Yerkes, another well-known psychologist, noted that in tests given young and old soldiers there was no difference in the intellectual powers of any of the soldiers, but the oldsters needed more time to complete the tests. Dr. Yerkes concluded that aged persons did not have the mental speed (just as they did not have the physical speed) of youngsters, but their mental abilities had not diminished with age.

Dr. Lorge said it was unfortunate that in industry and education it was often assumed that because one had a decline in muscular power and eyesight he also had a decline in intellectual power. "The age-old notion that men and women are not as 'good'—usually meaning mentally good—at forty, fifty, sixty, and even beyond, is wrong and unfair," said Dr. Lorge.

As Dr. Thorndike put it, "As the years advance, he

should, with quiet confidence, allow himself a little greater handicap for time. But I believe we can now assure every man and woman that, as the years go by, they do not need to allow themselves any *mental* handicap at all."

Regardless of what the medical and legal books say about senility and old age, *senility is not a result of age, but of starvation of the body and the brain.* With proper nutrition one will never be old mentally, provided, of course, he observes certain fundamental rules of health with which we are all familiar.

7. *A healthier endocrine glandular system will result from the diet.*
Dr. Tintera has said in several medical articles that the antihypoglycemia diet places the least possible amount of strain on the endocrines, particularly the adrenal glands, which are so important to our physical and mental health. Dr. Tintera has also shown us that weak and diseased adrenals have recuperative power; that is, the ability to become stronger and healthier glands, with the right kind of food.

8. *Adequate nutrition results in stronger bones.*
How tragic it is for an older person to have a fall and break a hip or even an arm or a leg! It is doubtful that some of these people will fully recover from the effects of a fall.

Osteoporosis, a structural weakness of the bones, is a disease of about one third of women over fifty years old. Men are a little less inclined to have osteoporosis, but older men seek medical care for the results of this disease daily.

A brittle bone can sometimes be fractured from some such simple movement as stooping, stepping down from a street curb, or missing a step on the stairs.

Backache is perhaps the commonest symptom of osteoporosis. New methods of measuring the density of bones now enable physicians to determine early in osteoporosis what percentage of the skeletal calcium is gone.

Dr. Jacob Bassan and associates, in *Annals of Internal Medicine* (March, 1963), stated, "Dietary studies in England and the United States indicate that patients with osteoporosis ingest less calcium in their diets as compared with nonosteoporotic contemporaries."

People advancing in years tend to ignore the calcium foods, eating instead cakes, cereals, and other foods with little or no food values. Some individuals who take an adequate amount of calcium have bones that do not harden. Vitamin D in the diet is necessary for the assimilation of calcium in the body. A deficiency of magnesium derived from the diet will make calcium absorption more difficult.

Some physicians feel that a low protein intake may be responsible for osteoporosis, and that the condition may be reversed by a high-protein diet. Drs. Grusin and Samuel, in an article in the *American Journal of Clinical Nutrition* (November-December, 1957), found that osteoporosis patients have a vitamin C deficiency. In 1961, Dr. W. K. Ramp, of the Veterans Administration Hospital at Lexington, Kentucky, and P. A. Thornton, of the University of Kentucky, used chickens for experimentation to determine what influence vitamin C had on the formation and the health of bones. All the chickens had vitamin D deficiency, but those fed vitamin C for two days had more minerals in their bones than did the chickens that were given no vitamin supplement.

Dr. James Greenwood, Jr., of the neurosurgery staff of Baylor University School of Medicine, gave a recent report to a symposium on spinal surgery at George Washington University Hospital on the value of ascorbic acid in the treatment of patients with a low back syndrome. Dr. Greenwood stated that since 1957 he had successfully treated more than five hundred disc injury patients with oral vitamin C. Admitting that physicians do not fully understand the metabolic chemistry resulting from high-dosage vitamin C, Dr. Greenwood pointed out that vitamin C is known to be intimately connected with the health and function of bone, cartilage, and connective tissue, all of which are involved in spinal disc difficulties.

Doctors believe that one reason the bones of our older people do not rebuild is that protein is no longer stimulated by lagging male and female hormones. Prescribing hormones is strictly the province of physicians; therefore we will not further discuss this cause of osteoporosis.

Dr. Daniel Bernstein warned in *Postgraduate Medicine* (October, 1963) that a lack of exercise can be harmful to bones. Many doctors talk about the "osteoporosis of disuse," which means that older people get brittle bones because they don't exercise enough.

There is no mystery about what osteoporosis is. It is a loss of calcium from the bones. Many published medical papers show that this disease is always accompanied by an insufficiency of calcium in the bloodstream. Unfortunately, too many old people (and sometimes their doctors) tend to consider the pains, disabilities, and illnesses of "senile osteoporosis," as the doctors call it, an inevitable and inescapable result of aging.

Milk is perhaps our best source of calcium. Some cannot tolerate milk, and for others it is very constipating. For those who can't take milk, bone meal is a very good substitute. As stated, vitamins A, C, and D, as well as foods containing phosphorus and magnesium, are needed for calcium to be properly absorbed and utilized in the body.

There are many ways in which a calcium deficiency manifests itself. If one is over sixty, and every time he touches or rubs the back of his hands or fingers against something, a purple spot appears which later turns black or brown, he may have a calcium deficiency. Here are some of the more or less common symptoms of calcium deficiency that in people past forty are often associated with "getting old," and that are mistakenly believed to be pains for which nothing can be done:

1. Cramps in the calf muscles of the leg, occurring during sleep or during exercise
2. Painful cramping of the feet and toes after going to bed
3. Contractions of the hands and fingers after use
4. Backaches
5. Insomnia
6. Dizziness
7. Nervous irritability and emotional instability
8. Brittle teeth with many cavities

9. Dermatitis of the scalp and face
10. Tremors of the fingers
11. Shortness of breath

It has long been known that calcium is necessary for normal regulation of the heartbeat. Many old people have been told that the lack of regular heart rhythm is nothing more than another symptom of old age.

Dr. Barry Fanburg presented a paper, "Cardiac Relaxing Factor" before a medical meeting in Boston on April 14, 1965, in which, in technical, medical language, he explained why it is necessary for the body to have an adequate supply of calcium for the heart muscles to function properly. Dr. Fanburg showed how calcium not only makes the heart beat strong and regularly, but is responsible for the ability of the heart to rest between beats.

Dr. Mildred Seelig, associate director of the Squibb Institute for Medical Research, writing in the *American Journal of Clinical Nutrition*, found that people living in the Orient who have adequate levels of magnesium in their diets, are free from arteriosclerosis. This physician called attention to the well-known medical fact that large amounts of calcium, protein, and vitamin D in the diet interfere with the absorption and retention of magnesium. Other researchers have shown that magnesium deficiency not only results in arteriosclerosis followed by atherosclerosis and coronary heart disease, but may result in various psychiatric disorders, such as convulsions and the less severe neuromuscular conditions.

Other physicians have recently discovered that the irregular heart rhythm of patients who have adequate calcium may be caused by coffee.

Dr. L. W. Cromwell reported to the Gerontological Society in San Francisco in September, 1953, that he had found calcium deficiency to be a cause of arthritic crippling in the aged.

It is easy to understand why cortisone (with its dangerous side effects) gives temporary relief to the arthritic sufferer. The excessive calcium of the bone joints, which nature has caused to be accumulated there for structural rigidity, is broken down by cortisone.

It follows from what we have said that the surest way *not* to have arthritis is always to follow a diet that has sufficient calcium and other minerals, and adequate vitamins.

9. *Good nutrition is essential to good health.*
Possibly a fourth or more of people over fifty accept pains and aches as inevitable, a burden for which nothing can be done except to "run to the doctor when the suffering becomes unbearable." What a fatalistic and foolish attitude!

Dr. M. Higuichi, of Japan, has done much research to show that the sex glands, particularly in older people, have need for vitamin C. Other physicians have shown that thiamine (vitamin $B_1$) and glutamic acid (one of the nonessential amino acids) cause the hormones of the male sex glands to continue to be produced until a very advanced age.

It seems that we will never know all of the wonderful health-giving properties of vitamin C. Surgeons know that this glamorous vitamin can prevent blood clots after operations—so vitamin C is prescribed before, during, and sometimes after surgery. Dr. Richard Bing, of Wayne State University, has found this vitamin of great value after myocardial infarction.

Dr. Boris Sokoloff, of Florida, believes that vitamin C "may be involved directly or indirectly in the fat metabolism and subsequently in the development of atherosclerosis."

Atherosclerosis is a chronic, usually progressive vascular disease, characterized by thickening and loss of elasticity of arterial walls, followed by secondary degenerative changes. In the past this disease has been attributed mostly to disordered fat metabolism.

Without discounting the importance of animal fat in causing atherosclerosis, researchers are now looking at sugar, bad dietary habits, lack of vitamins and minerals, poorly functioning adrenals, not enough exercise, and other causes of this degenerative disease, which is the forerunner of coronary diseases.

Dr. William Parsons, Jr., director of research at Jackson Clinic and Foundation, Madison, Wisc., has urged that a long-range test be given to ascertain the value of one of the B vitamins, $B_3$ (niacin, or nicotinic acid) in controlling high cholesterol in the bloodstream.

In the October, 1951, issue of *Nutrition Reviews*, it was stated that a reduction of serum cholesterol could be had with pectin. Pectin is found in the tissues of apples, pears, avocados, and other fruits and vegetables.

A two-year study by several Canadian doctors, reported in the *Canadian Medical Association Journal* for December 15, 1957, showed favorable effects of niacin (nicotinic acid) in reducing cholesterol. An article appearing in the *Medical Journal of Australia* in 1961 described vitamins A and D as having been successfully used to fight high cholesterol.

Many scientists believe that cancer prevention may occur as a result of good nutrition. Dr. E. Cheraskin and Dr. W. M. Ringsdorf, Jr., wrote in the journal *Cancer* (March 28, 1964) that in the course of testing forty apparently healthy policemen and firemen they found that twenty families with histories of cancer had either high or low blood sugar.

In October, 1964, Dr. Umberto Saffiotti, a Chicago pathologist, told the Ninth International Cancer Congress in Tokyo that he had succeeded in giving lung cancer to practically all animals tested by the same means that humans get lung cancer. He further stated that another group of similar animals after getting vitamin A were immune to cancer.

The July 10, 1951, *Journal of Nutrition* described the experiments on rats by the Sloan-Kettering Institute for Cancer. When the rats were fed known cancer-producing substances supplemented by a diet containing 15 per cent or more of brewer's yeast, none of them developed cancer. When the brewer's yeast was not given, or was less than 15 per cent of the feedings, the rats developed cancer. It will be noted that brewer's yeast is high in all of the B vitamins. From these experiments it was believed that the B vitamins, for some unknown reason, prevented the development of cancer in the rats.

Nobel Prize winner Dr. Otto Warburg, director of the

Max-Planck Institute for Cell Physiology in Berlin, in addressing a group of scientists in July, 1966, at Lindau, Germany, stated that in brewer's yeast and desiccated liver lie our best possible chances to avoid cancer.

The *German Tribune* for May 2, 1964, quoted Dr. Werner Grab, of the University of Giesen, as having said that vitamin C will inhibit cancer.

10. *A feeling of well-being and happiness is a reward of good nutrition.*

We have been told all of our lives that if we have good health—physical and mental—we have everything, and that if we have bad health, we have nothing. We are a rich nation; we have the finest hospitals and medical facilities, the best doctors, and all of the latest "wonder drugs."

The *New Jersey Business*, in June, 1960, quoted Dr. Winston Bostick, head of the Stevens Institute of Technology Physics Department, as follows, "There is a kind of unofficial conspiracy to picture Americans as the healthiest people in the world. Reliable evidence indicates we are not. America is fast becoming a nation of invalids and blame for this sorry state of health in a large part should be placed on our diet."

# 9

# Physical and mental
# health assured

When our doctor asks us how we feel, we say, "Fine," "Better today," "Not quite as strong," or some other phrase to express how we feel physically. If a physician should inquire about our mental health, we would be offended, thinking that our sanity was being questioned. Yet a state of mental health can, and often does, vary from day to day, as does physical health.

"I don't seem to be able to remember anything today," "I decided to work in the yard, since I wasn't able to concentrate at the office," "I felt so nervous and jumpy this morning I couldn't get any work done," and similar expressions indicative of the condition of mental health are continually heard, and, rightfully, are not considered of any great consequence.

The Freudian psychiatrists have done little or nothing to impress on the public the necessity for improving the mental health of all of us every day. One of them, called as a witness in court, frequently where a jury has to decide the issue involved, will testify that he does not recognize the words "sane" or "insane"; that these are legal, not medical, words. The witness will then go into a psychoanalytical lecture that soars completely over the heads of the judge and jurors; all they will remember of the doctor's testimony will be something about a person being able or not able to adjust to his environment.

The truth of the matter is that the standards of conduct prescribed by law for persons in both civil and criminal cases are not recognized by Freudians; consequently, their conclusions and deductions are of no value to judges and jurors in court.

Since the state of our mental health is determined in large measure by how well we are physically, let us see what we can do to improve both our physical and our mental health. Exercise is as beneficial as is good nutrition; in fact, one without the other won't keep us healthy.

The Committee on Aging of the American Medical Association, after a seven-year study, concluded: "Though staying in bed sometimes seems preferable to going to work, the body isn't engineered that way. It can stand a tremendous amount of abuse—years of it, in fact. Yet a week in bed will enfeeble even the strongest man, for without use the body falls into dilapidation like a vacant house. Unless we physically use our bodies, and we do it continually, we literally waste away in a fashion akin to aging. Muscles deteriorate and grow slack; bones become more porous and thus susceptible to damage; the circulatory system loses its tone and is more prone to atherosclerosis, and the heart loses some of its ability to cope with sudden tensions. All tissues, in fact, function better with physical stimulation, including the flow of vital chemicals secreted by our internal organs."

Dr. Joseph B. Wolffe, medical director of the Valley Forge Medical Center and Heart Hospital, speaking before the 44th Annual National Recreation Congress in Philadelphia, stated, "My presentation is from a heart specialist's point of view, although you doubtlessly would hear similar observations from a rheumatologist, orthopedic surgeon, or a neurologist.

"Leading cardiologists—both clinicians and researchers—of the American Heart Association and the National Health Institutes are in agreement that one of the factors contributing to atherosclerosis is lack of exercise. Atherosclerosis, widely prevalent disease of Western civilization and the most common form of 'hardening of the arteries,' is often regarded as a degenerative disease due to aging. While age is a factor, there are many old people in our country and vast numbers in countries like Yemen and parts of Africa and China, who are comparatively free from this disease.

"Atherosclerosis is characterized by accumulation of cholesterol and other fatty debris in the walls of the medium- and large-sized arteries which often plug the lumen, thus impeding or blocking the flow of blood. . . . In a study conducted at the Valley Forge Medical Center and Heart Hospital, we were impressed by a lack of clinical and laboratory evidence of atherosclerosis in a group of outstanding athletes who were continuing strenuous athletic endeavor well into their advancing years. Among them were old marathon runners up to sixty-seven years old. The cardiovascular efficiency of these active individuals was far superior to a comparative group of executives of a leading industrial firm of similar age level. This study confirms Mellerowicz's finding that the cardiovascular systems of old athletes who continued regular training were functionally equivalent to those of a much younger age group of the average population. . . .

"In a survey by Pomeroy and White, favorable results were reported on the influence of lifelong exercise in their study of ex-football players. Those who maintained a heavy exercise program throughout the postplaying years did not develop coronary heart disease. A study by Morris and his group in Great Britain showed that the number of heart attacks among sedentary workers, clerks, switchboard operators, and truck drivers was three times greater than among those engaged in physically active occupations—laborers, miners, transport workers, and farmers.

"The term 'athlete's heart,' which unfortunately still carries a connotation of abnormalcy, is a myth. There is no such clinical entity. . . . It is important to caution here that individuals who are unaccustomed to vigorous physical activity, or who have not exercised for a long time, should not indulge in strenuous physical effort without preparation. The man who has a heart attack while shoveling snow, whose only exercise prior to this vigorous exercise (since snow is heavy) was pushing a pen, a button, picking up a telephone receiver, or driving his car, only proves that he was 'soft.' His coronary arteries did not respond to a sudden need for meeting his unaccustomed demand. Many individuals are in very poor physical condition, but recreational exercise would condition them, re-educate their muscles, and reduce the number of heart attacks as well as sudden deaths. . . .

"The staff of the Valley Forge Medical Center and Heart Hospital insisted for more than a decade that there should be no elevator for their own or the patients' use. It is a three-story building. Eighty-five per cent of the patients suffer from either cardiac or vascular disease or both. Patients with acute heart failure or acute coronary thrombosis who should be at complete bed rest for a limited period are placed on the first floor. However, as soon as these patients are ambulatory and have been rehabilitated, they are encouraged to walk stairs.

"Stair walking involves all systems in the body. The body is carried upward by the skeletal muscles. Groups of muscles contract while their antagonists relax. . . . The heart and vessels are gradually strengthened. . . . One can walk at a pace which does not produce shortness of breath resulting from oxygen debt. . . . The nervous system plays its part in stair walking. The afferent and efferent nerves are flashing out impulses to improve the individual's co-ordination. . . .

"The endocrine system also plays a part even during such mild exercise as walking stairs. More corticosteroids are excreted at this time—these are the hormones that are used in the treatment of arthritis. This is another proof that physical movements are essential for the arthritic patient. . . .

"In all the years of my medical practice, I have yet to see any patient with heart disease die while walking stairs. I have known hundreds who died in bed. . . . The person—unless he is crippled—who avoids walking steps fails to take advantage of a safe 'built-in exercise.' I would exchange many fancy pills and injectable wonder drugs for a hospital recreation expert who would recondition or recreate these individuals whose bodies are wrecked as the result of the monotonous humdrum of life, the confinement indoors, and the lack of recreational physical activity."

Arthur Blumenfeld, in his excellent book *Heart Attack: Are You a Candidate?* said, "A moderate amount of exercise will be found sufficient to normalize blood cholesterol provided calories are watched and the diet fats are properly selected and consumed in moderation. . . . Exercise may be a potent factor in the prevention of heart attack, as evidence from many parts of the world shows."

Dr. Paul Dudley White, famous heart specialist, has said, "The chief danger of automobiles isn't from accidents but from the fact that they take people off their feet."

*Science News Letter* of April 28, 1962, told of the experiment of Dr. Lawrence Golding, of Kent State University. Dr. Golding studied forty-two white-collar, middle-aged workers whose cholesterol levels were all above normal. After a period of regular exercise, the average cholesterol level dropped from 261 to 195, and some individuals went from 300 down to 150 in cholesterol level readings. The men had no dietary restrictions, and most of them said their calorie consumption increased because of the exercise.

The *Journal of the American Medical Association* for October 5, 1957, stated, "The greatest value of exercise lies in its stimulating effect on endocrine gland activity, perhaps the thyroid in particular. . . ."

Physicians have noted that exercise, particularly walk-

* Quoted with permission from Alice K. Hand, administratrix of the estate of Joseph B. Wolffe, and from Valley Forge Medical Center and Heart Hospital, Morristown, Pennsylvania.

ing, causes the adrenal glands to secrete their hormones, one of which is cortisone, which stimulates mental activity and overcomes fatigue.

Exercise, especially walking, has always been known to be the best medicine for hypertension. Doctors say that a muscle tired from exercise is never a tense muscle. The wise physician will tell his patients to  good nutrition and adequate exercise, and not  tranquilizers, when they feel tense.

Dr. Vladimir Filatov in *My Path in Science* observed that glaucoma and other eye diseases are helped by long walks.

Dr. William Dock, of Brooklyn Veterans Administration Hospital, told the 114th Annual Convention of the American Medical Association that the heart starts to age soon after maturity, but that exercise staves off the wasting of heart muscles. "In general," said Dr. Dock, "the aging hearts of sedentary people near fifty years or older do not tolerate an overload."

Writing in *Clinical Nutrition* (December, 1966), Dr. Jean Mayer, Harvard University nutritionist, said, "It may well be that no currently available medical measure could be as beneficial as an increase in the amount of exercise taken by our population." In addition to heart diseases, Dr. Mayer cited diabetes and osteoporosis as resulting from our sedentary lives.

Dr. Charles Frank, of the Albert Einstein College, New York, recently explained that physical exercise increases one's ability to withstand a heart attack because the activity aids in the development of an increased number of blood vessels to the heart and between the arteries.

This cardiologist continued, "Even a little exercise seems to help. We don't have to be physical nuts, but it would help us to get off our bottoms once in a while."

A group of Canadian researchers challenged the present emphasis on the cholesterol–heart disease line in the January 9, 1965, *Canadian Medical Association Journal* by saying, "A theory of multiple causation seems more plausible than a dietary theory. . . . It may be easier to change the patterns of total physical activity of the population than to alter dietary habits."

Dr. Edward Bortz, an authority on aging at Philadelphia's Lankenau Hospital, recently said that various physical exercises for the aged will make old people feel better, "both physically and mentally" . . . . "Just as we have the 40,000-mile automobile tire, there is no reason why we can't have the 100-year hearts," commented Dr. Bortz.

Dr. Murray Miller, reporting to the American Therapeutic Society in San Francisco, recently stated that getting the aged to move around more may be all that is needed to cure senility. This Pennsylvania doctor said that getting these people out of bed, taking them by the arm and walking them, usually alleviated the symptoms of depression, torpor, and argumentativeness. Dr. Miller was very critical of the practice of putting old people to bed and writing a prescription for a tranquilizer. This, he said, resulted in a carbon dioxide buildup.

Dr. Herman Blumgart, of Harvard University, speaking on February 27, 1965, before the American College of Cardiology, said that exercise appears to offer the only nonsurgical means of treating atherosclerosis. Dr. Blumgart urged restraint in attempting surgery.

What type of exercise is best for us? Each person should select the kind of exercise that he likes best and that is best suited to him, whether it is swimming, golfing, tennis, bicycle riding, or any of the scores of other possibilities. Most doctors, in fact, believe that walking is the best form of exercise for most of us. Walking speeds up the body's metabolic processes and gently accelerates the action of the heart. Like all exercise, it makes the body firm and improves the appearance of the figure. It makes us more mentally alert, calms our emotions, and increases our enthusiasm for life.

A program of proper nutrition, as outlined in this book, combined with regular exercise will go a long way toward assuring all of us the "sound mind in a sound body" that has been man's ideal since antiquity.

*Appendix A*

**THE FAT-SOLUBLE VITAMINS**
**THE WATER-SOLUBLE VITAMINS**
**TABLE OF VITAMINS IN FOODS**

## THE FAT-SOLUBLE VITAMINS

*Vitamin A (also known as the anti-infective or anti-ophthalmic vitamin)*

This vitamin is found in most colored vegetables, many fruits, eggs, dairy products, margarines, liver, and fish-liver oils.

Vitamin A has these positive functions:

1. Builds resistance to infections, especially of the respiratory tract
2. Permits formation of visual purple in the eye, counteracting night blindness and weak eyesight
3. Promotes healthy skin
4. Helps maintain a healthy condition of the outer layers of many tissues and organs
5. Essential for pregnancy and lactation
6. Promotes growth and vitality
7. Increases longevity and delays senility

A deficiency of vitamin A may result in night blindness, increased susceptibility to infections, dry and scaly skin, lack of appetite and vigor, defective teeth having a thin and weak enamel, retarded growth, intestinal disorders, and general debility. Other organ systems affected by a deficiency of vitamin A are: digestive system, genitourinary system, special senses, and endocrine system.

An increased need for this vitamin occurs during infancy, pregnancy, and lactation.

An excess of vitamin A is stored in the body. Roughly 95 per cent of vitamin A reserves are stored in the liver.

*Vitamin D (also called the "sunshine vitamin," and Viosterol and Ergosterol)*

This vitamin is found in fish-liver oils, fats, eggs, milk, butter, and sunshine.

§153

The positive functions of vitamin D include:

1. Regulating the use of calcium and phosphorus in the body, and therefore necessary for the proper formation of bones and teeth

2. Essential for preventing rickets in children

3. Important for growth and development in infancy and childhood—a deficiency of vitamin D affects the bones and teeth, resulting in rickets in children and osteomalacia in adults

4. Necessary for growth and vigor of children

Deficiency of vitamin D results in these conditions:

a. Various skeletal deformities, as bowlegs, knock-knees, enlargement of the ends of the long bones, curvature of the spine, softening of the skull in infants and delayed closing of the anterior fontanelle

b. Swelling and beading of the ribs

c. Retarded growth and lack of vigor

d. Muscular weakness

e. Enlarged parathyroid glands

f. Low serum calcium and low body phosphorus; calcium and phosphorus retentions small or negative

g. Tooth decay

h. Rickets and osteomalacia

i. Various emotional and mental disturbances

Vitamin D excesses are stored chiefly in the liver; also in the skin, brain, spleen, and bones.

Hypervitaminosis D may result from an excessive and prolonged intake of this vitamin, some of the symptoms of hypervitaminosis being vomiting, headache, drowsiness, diarrhea, and loss of appetite for food. Occasionally we find a misguided mother who administers an abnormally high amount of vitamin D to a young child, which may result in serious impairment of health from deposits of excessive calcium in the heart, large vessels, renal tubules, and soft tissue.

*Vitamin E (also known as tocopherol)*

This vitamin is found in wheat germ, whole wheat, green leaves, vegetable oils, meat, eggs, whole-grain cereals, and margarine.

The positive functions of vitamin E are:

1. Antioxidant, which preserves easily oxydizable vitamins and unsaturated fatty acids in foods, mixtures, or the body

2. Necessary for normal reproduction and in helping to prevent sterility

3. Useful in helping prevent muscular dystrophy

4. Helpful in the treatment of threatened abortion

5. Prevents calcium deposits in blood vessel walls

6. Valuable in treatment of heart conditions and cardiovascular diseases generally

7. Useful in the prevention of some emotional and mental disorders

8. Necessary for growth and development of children

9. Successfully used in treating certain skin diseases

10. Acts as a regulator of the metabolism of the cell nucleus

11. Maintains normal permeability of capillaries

Some of the deficiency symptoms of this vitamin are: loss of reproductive powers, muscular disorders, fragility of red blood cells, nervousness, and general weakness.

*Vitamin K (also known as Menadione and the blood clotting vitamin)*

This vitamin is found in alfalfa and other green plants, soybean oils, and egg yolks.

The positive functions of vitamin K are:

1. Essential for the production of prothrombin, a substance which aids the blood in clotting

2. Important to combat hypoprothrombinemia in the newborn

A deficiency of vitamin K is caused by nutritional deficiencies, faulty intestinal synthesis and poor intestinal absorption, hepatic injury, and massive hemorrhages.

Deficiency symptoms are prolonged blood-clotting time and multiple hemorrhages, as in subcutaneous tissue, thymus, bladder, eye, adrenals, testis, kidney, and brain.

## THE WATER-SOLUBLE VITAMINS

*Thiamine (also known as vitamin $B_1$, thiamine chloride, the antineurotic and the antiberiberi vitamin)*

This vitamin is found in dried yeast, rice husks, whole wheat, oatmeal, peanuts, pork, milk, and most vegetables.

The positive functions of thiamine are:

1. Essential for normal functioning of nerve tissue

2. Necessary for good appetite, normal digestion, and gastrointestinal tonus

3. Needed for proper metabolism of carbohydrates and fats

4. Promotes growth

5. Aids muscular and heart development

6. Valuable in establishing good mental health

The deficiency symptoms of thiamine are:

a. In children, impaired growth

b. Mental depression and irritability

c. Loss of appetite, loss of weight, and various aches and pains

d. Constipation

e. Insomnia

f. Various forms of beriberi in advanced cases

Thiamine perhaps has more to do with a healthy nervous system than does any other vitamin. Loss of ankle and knee jerk reflexes, neuritis, muscular weakness in the feet, calves, and thighs are usually indicative of thiamine deficiency. Where the deficiency of this vitamin is marked, the subject may have mental instability, inability to remember, vague fears and uneasiness, and ideas of persecution.

Thiamine is not stored in the body; therefore it should be ingested each day for normal functioning.

## Riboflavin (also known as vitamin $B_2$)

This vitamin is found in liver, kidney, milk, yeast, cheese, and in most foods that contain thiamine.

The positive functions of riboflavin are:

1. Improves growth and promotes general health
2. Essential for healthy eyes, skin, and mouth
3. Important for respiration in poorly vascularized tissues

Deficiency symptoms of riboflavin are:

a. Cataracts

b. Corneal vascularization, cloudiness, and ulceration

c. Dimness of vision, burning and itching of the eyes, and impairment of vision

d. Congestion of the sclera

e. Abnormal pigmentation of the iris

f. Atrophy of the epidermis, sometimes with scaling

g. Lesions on lips and at corners of the mouth

h. Inflammation of tip and margin of the tongue, sometimes with a purplish color

i. "Sharkskin" appearance over the nose

j.  Impairment of wound-healing

k.  Degeneration of nervous tissues, resulting in incoordination, mental confusion, and loss of muscular strength in the arms and legs

*Niacin (also known as vitamin B₃ or nicotinic acid. This vitamin is sometimes manufactured as Niacinamide (Nicotinamide). Niacinamide is more generally used by doctors since it minimizes the burning, flushing, and itching of the skin that often occurs with niacin, or nicotinic acid)*

Liver, lean meat, whole wheat, yeast, green vegetables, and beans are good sources of vitamin $B_3$.

Some deficiency signs of this vitamin are:

1.  Pellagra, the most marked symptom being inflammation of the skin and tongue

2.  Gastrointestinal disturbance

3.  Dysfunction of the nervous system

4.  Mental depression and irritability

5.  Fatigue, headaches, and vague aches and pains

6.  Insomnia and general weakness

7.  Loss of appetite and loss of weight

8.  Neuritis

9.  Nausea, vomiting, and abdominal pains

10.  Burning hands and feet, pain in the calves, numbness, weakness, and difficulty in walking

11.  Diarrhea

12.  Mental symptoms ranging from loss of memory to stupor or mania

13.  Failing vision

14.  Prostration and death in extreme cases

A dietary deficiency of vitamin $B_3$ is usually accompanied by deficiencies of other members of the B-complex vitamin group, particularly thiamine, riboflavin, and pryidoxine.

Vitamin $B_3$ is especially important for the proper functioning of the nervous system. It promotes growth, maintains normal function of the gastrointestinal tract, is necessary for metabolism of sugar, and helps maintain normal skin condition.

We have already discussed the importance of this vitamin and others in the treatment of schizophrenia.

While not always true, generally it may be said that the functions and deficiency symptoms of all the members of the B-complex vitamin group are somewhat similar.

*Pyridoxine (also known as vitamin $B_6$)*

This vitamin is found in meat, fish, wheat germ, egg yolk, cantaloupe, cabbage, yeast, and milk.

The positive functions of pyridoxine are:

1. Aids in food assimilation and in protein and fat metabolism
2. Prevents various nervous and skin disorders
3. Needed for the utilization of amino acids

Deficiency symptoms of pyridoxine are loss of appetite, nausea, vomiting, lethargy, and dermatitis about the eyes, in the eyebrows, and at the angles of the mouth.

Mental confusion, numbness of the hands and feet, impairment of vibration and position sense are also deficiency signs.

*Biotin (one of the newly discovered members of the B-complex vitamin family)*

This vitamin is found in yeast and is present in at least minute quantities in every living cell.

The positive functions of biotin are:
1. Promotion of growth
2. Related to metabolism of fats
3. Essential in the conversion of certain amino acids

A deficiency of biotin may be caused by improper diet and impaired intestinal synthesis of microorganisms. Researchers have found that raw egg white fed to animals will destroy biotin.

Biotin deficiency symptoms are:
1. Exhaustion and drowsiness
2. Muscle pains and loss of appetite
3. A type of anemia complicated by skin disease

In addition to foods containing biotin, this vitamin is synthesized by intestinal flora.

*Pantothenic acid (also known as calcium pantothenate, another member of the B-complex family)*

This vitamin is found in liver, kidney, yeast, wheat, bran, peas, and crude molasses.

The positive functions of pantothenic acid are:
1. Necessary for normal digestive processes
2. Required for synthesis of antibodies
3. Helps to build body cells and to maintain normal skin, growth, and development of central nervous system

Pantothenic acid is essential for all living organisms, including man, and was formerly called "the anti-gray hair vitamin," as it was believed to be a factor in restoring gray hair to its original color. This function of the vitamin has not been substantiated.

Deficiency signs of the vitamin are:
1. Retarded growth
2. Painful and burning feet

3. Digestive disturbances
4. Skin abnormalities
5. Dizzy spells
6. Diarrhea with bloody stools
7. Mental and emotional disturbances—subjects becoming discontented, quarrelsome, irascible, easily upset, and antagonistic
8. Rapid heart rate on exertion
9. Epigastric distress and constipation
10. Numbness and tingling of hands and feet
11. Weakness of the extensor muscles of the fingers

This vitamin is related to the utilization of other vitamins, especially riboflavin, and depends also on the availability of folic acid and biotin. It is involved in adrenal function.

*Folic acid (another member of the B-complex family)*

This vitamin is found in yeast, liver, kidney, and dark-green leafy vegetables.

The positive functions of folic acid are:
1. Essential to the formation of red blood cells by its action on the bone marrow
2. Aids in protein metabolism and contributes to normal growth
3. Action related to that of ascorbic acid (vitamin C).

Deficiency symptoms of the vitamin are:
1. Nutritional macrocytic anemia
2. Endocrine disturbance

*Vitamin $B_{12}$ (also known as the "red vitamin," and a member of the B-complex family)*

This vitamin comes from liver, beef, pork, eggs, milk, and cheese. It is also formed by bacterial synthesis.

The positive functions of vitamin $B_{12}$ are:

1. Aids in the formation and regeneration of red blood cells, thus preventing anemia
2. Promotes growth and increased appetites in children
3. Acts as a tonic for adults
4. Improves mental health

Deficiency of vitamin $B_{12}$ leads to these symptoms:

a. Nutritional and pernicious anemia
b. Poor appetite and growth failure in childhood
c. Tiredness
d. Nervousness, mental confusion, and, in some instances, irrational talk and conduct.

Vitamin $B_{12}$ content is high in the organ meats, as liver, kidney, etc. It is medium in fish and the muscle meats and low in milk, yeast, soybeans, wheat, and corn.

*Ascorbic acid (also known as cevitamic acid and vitamin C)*

This vitamin is found in citrus fruits, berries, greens, cabbages, and peppers. It is easily destroyed by cooking.

The positive functions of vitamin C are:

1. Necessary for healthy teeth, gums, and bones
2. Strengthens all connective tissue
3. Promotes wound healing
4. Prevents blood clots during and following surgery
5. Promotes capillary integrity and prevents permeability
6. Important factor in maintaining sound physical and mental health
7. May be involved in the absorption and utilization of dietary iron and the maintenance of normal blood hemoglobin levels
8. Related to the metabolism of certain amino acids
9. A relationship may exist between vitamin C and the

production of adrenalcortical hormones in view of the high concentration of this vitamin in the adrenals

10. Blood vitamin A levels are correlated with plasma ascorbic acid contents

11. Probably a component of a reversible oxidation-reduction system in the body, acting as a hydrogen transporter

12. Promotes knitting of bones following fractures

13. Prevents scurvy

14. Important for healthy skin and eyes

TABLE OF VITAMINS IN FOODS

*VITAMIN D IN FOODS*
*A—micrograms; B—International Units: per 100 g.*
*edible portion*

|  | A | B |
|---|---|---|
| Beef steak | 0.33 | 13 |
| Beet greens | 0.004 | 0.2 |
| Bread, vitamin D | 1.7 | 68 |
| Butter | 2.3 | 92 |
| Cabbage | 0.005 | 0.2 |
| Carrot tops | 0.075 | 3 |
| Cheese | 0.83 | 33 |
| Cod-liver oil | 250 | 10,000 |
| Corn oil | 0.22 | 9 |
| Cream | 0.42 | 17 |
| Crisco | 0.22 | 9 |
| Egg yolk | 6.6 | 265 |
| Halibut-liver oil | 3500 | 140,000 |
| Herring, canned | 8.2 | 330 |
| Liver, beef, raw | .85 | 34 |
| Liver, lamb, raw | .45 | 18 |
| Liver, pork, raw | 1.10 | 44 |
| Liver, veal | 0.24 | 9.6 |
| Mackerel, fresh, raw | 27.7 | 1100 |
| Milk, whole | 0.11 | 4.4 |
| Milk, vitamin D | 1.1 | 44 |
| Pilchards, canned | 18.6 | 745 |
| Salmon, raw | 7.4 | 297 |
| Salmon, canned | 7.8 | 314 |
| Sardines, canned | 34.5 | 1380 |
| Shrimp | 3.75 | 150 |
| Spinach | .005 | 0.2 |
| Tuna | 5-8 | 200-320 |

*VITAMIN E*
TOCOPHEROL CONTENT OF FOODS
*mg. per 100 g. of fresh material*

|  | Total | *Alpha* |
|---|---|---|
| Apples | 0.74 | 0.72 |
| Bacon | 0.53 | 0.44 |
| Bananas | 0.40 | 0.37 |
| Beans, dry navy | 3.60 | 0.10 |
| Beef liver | 1.40 | 1.40 |
| Beef steak | 0.63 | 0.47 |
| Butter | 2.40 | ----- |
| Carrots | 0.45 | 0.45 |
| Celery | 0.48 | 0.46 |
| Chicken | 0.25 | 0.21 |
| Coconut oil | 8.30 | 3.60 |
| Cornmeal, yellow | 1.70 | 0.84 |
| Corn oil | 87 | 7 |
| Cottonseed oil | 90 | 56 |
| Eggs, whole | 2.00 | 1.16 |
| Grapefruit | 0.26 | 0.25 |
| Haddock | 0.39 | 0.35 |
| Lamb chops | 0.77 | 0.62 |
| Lettuce | 0.50 | 0.29 |
| Margarine | 54 | 28 |
| Oatmeal | 2.10 | 1.94 |
| Onions | 0.26 | 0.21 |
| Oranges | 0.24 | 0.23 |
| Peanut oil | 22 | 11 |
| Peas, green | 2.10 | 0.10 |
| Potatoes, sweet | 4.0 | 4.0 |
| Potatoes, white | 0.06 | ----- |
| Pork chops | 0.71 | 0.63 |
| Rice, brown | 2.40 | 1.20 |

*VITAMIN E (Cont.)*

|  | Total | *Alpha* |
|---|---|---|
| Soybean oil | 140 | 10 |
| Tomatoes | 0.36 | 0.27 |
| Turnip greens | 2.30 | 2.24 |

*VITAMIN K*
DIETARY SOURCES
*micrograms per 100 g. of edible portion*

| | | | |
|---|---|---|---|
| Alfalfa | 425–850 | Potatoes | 20 |
| Cabbage | 250 | Soybeans | 190 |
| Cauliflower | 275 | Spinach | 334 |
| Carrots | 10 | Strawberry | 13 |
| Corn | 10 | Tomato, green | 49 |
| Liver, pork | 115–230 | Tomato, ripe | 24 |
| Mushrooms | 7 | Wheat | 36 |
| Oats | 75 | Wheat bran | 80 |
| Peas | 7 | Wheat germ | 37 |

*PYRIDOXINE (VITAMIN B$_6$)*
DIETARY SOURCES
*micrograms per 100 g. of edible portion*

| | | | |
|---|---|---|---|
| Apple | 26 | Brains, beef | 160 |
| Asparagus, cnd. | 30 | Cabbage | 120–290 |
| Banana | 320 | Cantaloupe | 36 |
| Barley | 320–560 | Cauliflower | 20 |
| Beans, green, cnd. | 32 | Carrot, raw | 120–220 |
| | | Cheese | 98 |
| Beef | 230–320 | Cod | 340 |
| Beer | 50–60 | Corn, cnd. | 68 |
| Beet greens | 37 | Corn, yellow | 360–570 |

## PYRIDOXINE (VITAMIN B₆) (Cont.)

| | | | |
|---|---|---|---|
| Corn grits ____ | 200 | Salmon, cnd. __ | 450 |
| Cottonseed | | Salmon, fresh _ | 590 |
| meal _____ | 1310 | Sardines, cnd. _ | 280 |
| Eggs, fresh ___ | 22–48 | Soybeans _____ | 710–1200 |
| Flounder _____ | 100 | Spinach, cnd. __ | 60 |
| Grapefruit | | sections ____ | 17–24 |
| juice _____ | 8–18 | Halibut _____ | 110 |
| Grapefruit | | Heart, beef ___ | 200–290 |
| Milk, whole ___ | 54–110 | Honey _____ | 4–27 |
| Milk, dry _____ | 330–820 | Kidney, beef __ | 350–990 |
| Milk, dry skim_ | 550 | Lamb _____ | 250–370 |
| Molasses, | | Lemon juice __ | 35 |
| blackstrap __ | 2000–2490 | Lettuce _____ | 71 |
| Oats, rolled ___ | 93–150 | Liver, beef ____ | 600–710 |
| Onions _____ | 63 | Liver, calves __ | 300 |
| Orange juice, | | Liver, pork ___ | 290–590 |
| cnd. _____ | 16–31 | Malt extract __ | 540 |
| Orange juice, | | Strawberries __ | 44 |
| fresh _____ | 18–56 | Tomatoes, cnd. | 710 |
| Peaches, cnd.__ | 16 | Tuna, cnd. ____ | 440 |
| Peanuts _____ | 300 | Veal _____ | 280–410 |
| Peas, cnd. ____ | 46 | Watermelon __ | 33 |
| Peas, dry _____ | 160–330 | Wheat bran ___ | 1380–1570 |
| Pork _____ | 330–680 | Wheat germ __ | 850–1600 |
| Potato _____ | 160–250 | White flour ___ | 380–600 |
| Raisins _____ | 94 | Yams _____ | 320 |
| Rice, whole ___ | 1030 | Yeast, bakers' _ | 620–700 |
| Rice, white ___ | 340–450 | Yeast, brewers' | |
| Rye _____ | 300–370 | dry _____ | 4000–5700 |

*BIOTIN*
DIETARY SOURCES
*micrograms per 100 g. of edible portion*

| | | | |
|---|---|---|---|
| Bananas | 4 | Milk | 5 |
| Beans, dried lima | 10 | Molasses | 9 |
| Beef | 4 | Mushrooms | 16 |
| Carrots | 2 | Onions, dry | 4 |
| Cauliflower | 17 | Oysters | 9 |
| Cheese | 2 | Peas, fresh | 2 |
| Chicken | 5–10 | Peas, dried | 18 |
| Chocolate | 32 | Peanuts, roasted | 39 |
| Corn | 6 | Pork, bacon | 7 |
| Eggs, whole fresh | 25 | Pork, muscle | 2–5 |
| Filberts | 16 | Salmon | 5 |
| Grapefruit | 3 | Spinach | 2 |
| Halibut | 8 | Strawberries | 4 |
| Hazel nuts | 14 | Tomatoes | 2 |
| Liver, beef | 100 | Wheat, whole | 5 |

*PANTOTHENIC ACID*
DIETARY SOURCES
*micrograms per 100 g. of edible portion*

| | | | |
|---|---|---|---|
| Beans, dried lima | 830 | Broccoli | 1400 |
| | | Cauliflower | 920 |
| Beef, brain | 2140–2860 | Cheese | 350–960 |
| Beef, heart | 2100–2470 | Chicken | 530–900 |
| Beef, kidney | 3400 | Eggs | 2700 |
| Beef, liver | 5660–8180 | Lamb | 600 |
| Beef, muscle | 1100 | Lamb, kidney | 4330 |
| Bread, whole wheat | 570 | Milk, whole | 290 |
| | | Mushrooms | 1700 |
| Bread, white | 400 | Oats | 1300 |

*PANTOTHENIC ACID (Cont.)*

| | | | |
|---|---|---|---|
| Oranges _____ | 340 | Pork, muscle _ | 470–1500 |
| Oysters _____ | 490 | Potatoes, Irish | 400–650 |
| Peas, fresh __ | 600–1040 | Potatoes, | |
| Peas, dried __ | 2800 | sweet _____ | 940 |
| Peanuts, | | Salmon _____ | 660–1100 |
| roasted ___ | 2500 | Soy beans ___ | 1800 |
| Pork, bacon__ | 280–980 | Veal chops ___ | 110–260 |
| Pork, ham ___ | 340–660 | Wheat, whole | 1300 |
| Pork, kidney _ | 3140 | Wheat, germ_ | 2000 |
| Pork, liver ___ | 5880–7300 | Wheat, bran _ | 2400 |

*FOLIC ACID CONTENT OF FOODS*
*micrograms per 100 g. of edible portion*

MEAT, EGGS

| | Total Folic Acid | Free Folic Acid |
|---|---|---|
| *Beef* | | |
| Round steak _____ | 7–17 | 6.7 |
| Chuck _____ | 15.2 | _____ |
| Hamburger _____ | 5.0 | 3.6 |
| Heart _____ | 3.1 | _____ |
| Kidney _____ | 58.4 | _____ |
| Liver _____ | 294 | _____ |
| Sweetbreads _____ | 22.8 | _____ |
| *Lamb* | | |
| Stew meat _____ | 1.9 | .4 |
| Leg _____ | 3.3 | _____ |
| Liver _____ | 276 | _____ |
| *Pork* | | |
| Liver _____ | 221 | _____ |
| Loin _____ | 2.4 | .2 |

## FOLIC ACID CONTENT OF FOODS (Cont.)

|  | Total Folic Acid | Free Folic Acid |
|---|---|---|
| Ham, smoked | 7.8 | .3 |
| Sausage | 12.5 | .5 |
| *Poultry* |  |  |
| Chicken, dark | 2.8 | ------- |
| Chicken, white | 3.1 | ------- |
| Chicken, liver | 377 | ------- |
| Turkey | 3–15 | 4–12 |
| *Eggs* |  |  |
| Whole | 5.1 | ------- |
| White | .6 | ------- |
| Yolk | 12.9 | ------- |
| **NUTS** |  |  |
| Almonds | 45.7 | ------- |
| Brazil nuts | 4.5 | ------- |
| Coconuts | 27.6 | ------- |
| Filberts | 66.6 | ------- |
| Peanuts | 56.6 | ------- |
| Pecans | 27.0 | ------- |
| Walnuts | 77.0 | ------- |
| **VEGETABLES (FRESH)** |  |  |
| Asparagus | 89–142 | 59.6 |
| Beans, Lima | 10–56 | 5.6 |
| Beans, Lima, dry | 103 | 16–36 |
| Beans, snap | 13–56 | 10.7 |
| Beans, Navy, dry | 129 | 11–33 |
| Beans, wax | 15–39 | ------- |

## FOLIC ACID CONTENT OF FOODS (Cont.)

|  | Total Folic Acid | Free Folic Acid |
|---|---|---|
| Beets | 13.5 | 3.3 |
| Broccoli | 33.9 | 8–14 |
| Brussels sprouts | 27.1 | 11.7 |
| Cabbage | 6–42 | 3.1 |
| Carrots | 8 | 3.2 |
| Cauliflower | 29.1 | 8.5 |
| Celery | 7.2 | 2.5 |
| Corn, sweet | 9–70 | 5 |
| Cucumbers | 6.7 | 3.8 |
| Egg plant | 5–15 | 3.8 |
| *Greens* | | |
| Beet | 20–50 | 23.8 |
| Chicory | 30 | 4.9 |
| Endive | 27–63 | ------- |
| Escarole | 25.8 | ------- |
| Kale | 50.9 | 31.0 |
| Mustard | 17–38 | ------- |
| Parsley | 42.9 | ------- |
| Spinach | 49–115 | 31–110 |
| Swiss chard | 32–64 | 5 |
| Turnip | 83.4 | 39.1 |
| Water cress | 47.6 | ------- |
| Kohlrabi | 10.1 | ------- |
| Lentils, dry | 99 | 24.5 |
| Lettuce | 4–54 | 2–12 |
| Mushrooms | 14–29 | 20.5 |
| Okra | 24.1 | ------- |
| Onions | | |
| Green, with tops | 12.6 | ------- |

## FOLIC ACID CONTENT OF FOODS (Cont.)

| | Total Folic Acid | Free Folic Acid |
|---|---|---|
| Mature | 6–14 | ------- |
| Parsnips | 8–37 | 7.6 |
| Peas | 5–35 | 4–15 |
| Peas, dry split | 22 | 6.2 |
| Peppers, green | 4–11 | 1.5 |
| Potatoes, peeled | 4–12 | 2–3 |
| Potato peels | 14.4 | 6.6 |
| Potatoes, whole | 2–135 | 3.3 |
| Pumpkin | 5–10 | 4.6 |
| Radishes | 3–10 | 2.7 |
| Rutabagas | 3–7 | 3.3 |
| Soy beans, dry | 1.92 | 91.6 |
| Squash | | |
| Acorn | 16.7 | 10.1 |
| Crookneck | 7–16 | 5 |
| Zucchini | 10.8 | ------- |
| Sweet potatoes | 5–19 | ------- |
| Tomatoes | 2–16 | 4 |
| Turnips | 4.3 | ------- |

FRUIT

| | Total Folic Acid | Free Folic Acid |
|---|---|---|
| Apples | .5 | ------- |
| Apricots | 3.6 | 4 |
| Apricots, dried | 4.7 | 1.6 |
| Avocados | 6–57 | 17.6 |
| Bananas | 9.6 | 6.1 |
| *Berries* | | |
| Blackberries | 6–18 | 14.5 |
| Blueberries | 7.6 | 2.7 |

## FOLIC ACID CONTENT OF FOODS (Cont.)

|  | Total Folic Acid | Free Folic Acid |
|---|---|---|
| Cranberries | 1.7 | .5 |
| Red raspberries | 5.1 | 3.2 |
| Strawberries | 5.3 | 1.6 |
| Cantaloupes | 3–8 | 8.8 |
| Cherries, Bing | 6.5 | 3.0 |
| Dates, dry | 24.7 | 10.0 |
| Figs | 6.7 | ------- |
| Figs, dry | 7–14 | 4.2 |
| Grapefruit | 2.7 | 1.4 |
| Grapes, green | 4.5 | 1.4 |
| Grapes, red | 4.9 | 3.1 |
| Honeydew melon | 4.9 | 4.1 |
| Lemons | 7.4 | 2.4 |
| Limes | 4.6 | 2.6 |
| Oranges | 5.1 | 2.4 |
| Orange juice | 4.8 | ------- |
| Peaches, yellow | 2.3 | .6 |
| Pears | 2.5 | .7 |
| Pineapple | .8–6 | 1.5 |
| Plums, red | .6–3 | .7 |
| Plums, yellow | 1.2 | .3 |
| Prunes, dry | 5.4 | 3.5 |
| Rhubarb | 2.5 | .5 |
| Tangerines | 7.4 | 1.3 |
| Watermelon | .6 | .3 |

### CEREALS AND OTHER GRAIN PRODUCTS

*Breads*

| Cracked wheat | 27 | ------- |
|---|---|---|

## FOLIC ACID CONTENT OF FOODS (Cont.)

|  | Total Folic Acid | Free Folic Acid |
|---|---|---|
| Rye | 19.8 | ------- |
| Vienna | 11.2 | ------- |
| White | 15 | ------- |
| *Breakfast Cereals* | | |
| Cornflakes | 5.5 | 2.8 |
| Cornmeal | 6.5 | 2.4 |
| Corn and soya | 80.1 | 14.2 |
| Oats, ready to eat | 22.5 | 6.3 |
| Oatmeal | 30.5 | 7.8 |
| Wheat bran | 100 | 24–47 |
| Wheat farina | 13.6 | 6.2 |
| Wheat, shredded | 29–87 | 8–28 |
| *Flour* | | |
| Cake | 6.6 | ------- |
| Rye | 18.0 | ------- |
| White, enriched | 8.1 | ------- |
| Whole wheat | 38 | ------- |
| *Grains* | | |
| Barley | 50 | 21.0 |
| Corn, yellow | 23.6 | 5.0 |
| Oats, white | 23–66 | 13–26 |
| Rice, brown | 22 | 10.9 |
| Rye | 34.4 | 13.8 |
| Wheat | 27–51 | .8–30 |

### MILK AND CHEESE

| *Milk* | | |
|---|---|---|
| Buttermilk | 11.1 | ------- |
| Evaporated milk | .7 | ------- |

## FOLIC ACID CONTENT OF FOODS (Cont.)

|  | Total Folic Acid | Free Folic Acid |
|---|---|---|
| *Cheese* | | |
| Cheddar | 15.5 | ------- |
| Cottage | 21–46 | ------- |
| Processed | 11.1 | ------- |

SOURCE: The foregoing tables reproduced from *Nutritional Data*, fifth edition, second revised printing, 1964, with permission of H. J. Heinz Company, © 1964.

*Appendix B*

## DIETARY LEVELS OF HOUSEHOLDS IN THE UNITED STATES, SPRING 1965
*Report of the U.S. Department*
*of Agriculture*

DIETARY LEVELS OF HOUSEHOLDS IN THE
UNITED STATES, SPRING 1965:

A Preliminary Report, *by Consumer and Food Economics Research Division, Agricultural Research Service, United States Department of Agriculture*

## Summary

A survey of the food consumption of a nationwide sample of 7,500 households made in the spring of 1965 shows that:
— Half of the households had diets that met the allowances for all nutrients. These diets were rated "good."
— The other half of the households had diets that failed to meet the allowances for one or more nutrients. Calcium, vitamin A value, and ascorbic acid were the nutrients most often found to be below allowances.
— About one-fifth of the diets provided less than two-thirds of the allowances for one or more nutrients. These diets were rated "poor."
— Little difference was found in the proportion of households with diets below the allowances for one or more nutrients in the four regions—Northeast, North Central, South, and West. Southern households spent less for food than households in other regions, but they had a greater nutritional return for each dollar spent.
— Similar proportions of urban and rural households had diets below the allowances for one or more nutrients. More rural than urban diets were below allowances for vitamin A value and ascorbic acid. But for most of the other nutrients studied, more urban than rural diets were below allowances.
— At each successively higher level of income, a greater percentage of households had diets that met allowances. High income of itself, however, did not insure good diets. More than one-third, 37 percent, of the households with incomes of

$10,000 and over had diets that were below the allowances for one or more nutrients.

– Almost two-thirds, 63 percent, of the households with incomes under $3,000 had diets that did not meet the allowances for one or more nutrients.

– Over one-third, 36 percent, of the households with incomes under $3,000 had poor diets. At this income level poor diets occurred most frequently among urban households in the North Central and rural households in the South.

– Fewer households had good diets in 1965 than in 1955— 50 percent in 1965 and 60 percent in 1955. The proportion with poor diets increased over the 10-year period from about 15 percent in 1955 to 20 percent in 1965. Decreased use of milk and milk products and vegetables and fruit, the main sources of calcium, ascorbic acid, and vitamin A value, was chiefly responsible for these changes in dietary levels.

INTRODUCTION

Amounts of food used in U.S. households in the spring of 1965 were sufficient, on the average, to provide diets meeting the Recommended Dietary Allowances set by the Food and Nutrition Board of the National Academy of Sciences-National Research Council for calories and protein; for the minerals, calcium and iron; and for the vitamins, vitamin A value, thiamine, riboflavin, and ascorbic acid.

Averages, however, conceal the great variation in the amounts of food used by different households. Half of the households had diets that furnished the recommended allowances for all of the nutrients studied, and the other half had diets that failed to meet the allowance for one or more nutrients. Ninety percent or more of all the household diets supplied the recommended allowances for protein, iron, thiamine, and riboflavin; nearly 75 percent supplied the allowances for vitamin A value and ascorbic acid; and 70 percent supplied the allowance for calcium. Of every 10 households with diets that did not supply the allowances for one or more nutrients, roughly four were short in only one nutrient, three in two, and another three in three or more.

The recommended allowances are daily calorie and nutrient intakes judged by scientists of the Food and Nutrition Board to be adequate for maintaining good nutrition in essentially all healthy persons in the United States under current conditions of living. The allowances provide a margin of sufficiency above average physiological requirements for each nutrient, but not for calories, to cover variations in needs among healthy persons.

The Food and Nutrition Board explains, however, that: "If the recommended allowances are used as reference standards for interpreting records of food consumption, it should not be assumed that food practices are necessarily poor or that malnutrition exists because the recommendations are not completely met."

In this report a diet is termed "good" when the nutritive value of the total food used by the household equaled or exceeded the recommended allowance for each of the seven nutrients for all the members of the household. By this criterion, one-half of the household diets rated "good."

In the other half of the households, some diets provided nutrients in amounts well below the allowances. When a diet supplied less than two-thirds of the recommended allowances for one or more nutrients, it was rated "poor." Two-thirds of the allowance for any nutrient is considered a level below which diets could be nutritionally inadequate for some individuals over an extended period of time.

One-fifth of the household diets rated poor. Only 1 or 2

percent of the diets supplied less than two-thirds of the allowance for protein, iron, thiamine, and riboflavin. However, 8 percent were this low in calcium, 10 percent in vitamin A value, and 13 percent in ascorbic acid. The nutrient shortages were associated with relatively low consumption of milk and milk products and vegetables and fruit, the principal food sources of calcium, vitamin A value, and ascorbic acid. On the average, about 60 percent of the calcium in the diets was supplied by milk and milk products, while half the vitamin A value and almost all the ascorbic acid were supplied by vegetables and fruit.

REGIONAL DIFFERENCES

Approximately half of the households in each region had diets that did not meet the allowances for all nutrients—52 percent in the North Central and South, 48 percent in the West, and 47 percent in the Northeast.

In all four regions, diets were most frequently below the allowances for calcium, vitamin A value, and ascorbic acid. More diets in the North Central and South than in the other regions did not meet the allowances for vitamin A value and ascorbic acid.

The regional differences in percent of diets below allowances for vitamin A value and ascorbic acid reflect the lower use per person of vegetables and fruit by North Central and Southern families than other families. Despite lower average consumption of milk, cream, and cheese in the South, percentage of diets in this region below the allowances for calcium was about the same as in other regions. The kinds and quantities of grain products used by Southern families supplied more calcium to their diets than that used by families in other regions.

The percentage of calcium contributed by milk, cream, and cheese plus flour, cereals, and bakery products was about the same for the South as for other regions, slightly under 80 percent.

Southern households used less expensive foods and had better diets for the money value of their foods than the households in other regions—$7.92 per person per week in the South compared with $8.67 in the North Central, $9.35 in the West, and $9.77 in the Northeast. A dollar's worth of food in the South provided more calories and more of each nutrient than a dollar's worth in other regions.

RURAL-URBAN DIFFERENCES

About as many urban as rural farm and nonfarm households had diets that did not meet the allowances for one or more nutrients. Slightly more rural than urban diets did not meet the allowances for vitamin A value and ascorbic acid. Greater use by urban families of dark-green and deep-yellow vegetables, rich in vitamin A value, and citrus fruits, rich in ascorbic acid, contributed to these differences.

Slightly more urban than farm diets did not meet the calcium, iron, and thiamine allowances. Consumption of more milk, cream, and cheese by farm than urban families (4.20 compared with 4.05 quarts, calcium equivalent, per person per week) and more grain products (3.44 compared with 2.46 pounds, flour equivalent) accounted for the additional amounts of these nutrients for farm families. The percentages of rural nonfarm households with diets not meeting the allowances for these three nutrients were between those of urban and farm households.

When households were classified by urbanization within the regions, other differences appeared. Diets that did not meet the allowances were most frequent in the Northeast and the West, among rural nonfarm households; in the North Central, among urban households; and in the South, among rural farm households.

DIFFERENCES BY INCOME

Dietary adequacy, as measured by the percentage of household diets meeting the allowances for all seven nutrients, was related to income. At each successively higher level of income, a greater percentage of households had diets that met the allowances.

High income alone did not insure good diets. More than one-third of the households with incomes of $10,000 and over had diets that did not meet the allowances for one or more nutrients.

Differences in the kinds of foods used at different income levels were not the result of income alone. Such differences undoubtedly reflect the many factors involved in food preferences and other family characteristics.

Low-income households had greater returns in calories and nutrients per food dollar, on the average, than households with high incomes.

COMPARISON WITH 1955

Average amounts of some foods used in 1965 were appreciably different from the amounts used in 1955, when the USDA made a similar nationwide food consumption survey. The principal differences were the increased use in 1965 of bakery products and meat, poultry, and fish, and decreased use of milk and milk products, flour and cereals, and vegetables and fruit. (See earlier preliminary report, ARS 62–16, August 1967.)

In both 1955 and 1965 fewer diets met the allowances for calcium, vitamin A value, and ascorbic acid than for other nutrients. Proportions of diets meeting the allowances in 1965 were lower for these three nutrients than in 1955.

Good diets, those meeting allowances for all seven nutrients, were found in 5 of every 10 households surveyed in 1965 and in 6 of every 10 households in 1955. About 20 percent of the diets in 1965 were poor, those with less than two-thirds of the allowance for one or more of the nutrients, and about 15 percent in 1955.

Increased consumption of milk or other worthwhile sources of calcium, vegetables, and fruit is needed to improve the household diets not meeting the allowances. High incomes and high expenditures for food are related to good diets, but neither guarantees them. Awareness of the foods that make up a good diet, a desire to choose these foods, and sufficient money to buy adequate food must become more universal if most U.S. households are to have good diets.

SCOPE AND NATURE OF SURVEY

In addition to the 7,500 housekeeping households surveyed in the spring of 1965, 2,500 households were surveyed in each of the other three seasons—summer 1965, fall 1965, and winter 1965. In all, a total of 15,000 households were surveyed.

The Department of Agriculture has made similar nation-wide surveys of household food consumption in 1936, 1942, 1948 (urban only), and 1955. The 1965–66 survey is the first to include nationwide data on diets of individual family members and on household food consumption for all seasons of the year. Results on these aspects will be reported in later publications.

*Appendix C*

## TREATMENT OF SCHIZOPHRENIA

## TREATMENT OF SCHIZOPHRENIA

*From* How to Live With Schizophrenia, *by Dr. Abram Hoffer and Dr. Humphry Osmond, with permission from University Books, New Hyde Park, N. Y.,* © *1966.*

TREATMENT PROGRAM

Our treatment program is divided into three phases, each phase depending on how long you have been sick, and how your schizophrenia responds to treatment. We will describe our program as if you, the reader, are a patient on the other side of our desk seeking help.

PHASE ONE TREATMENT

You have Phase One schizophrenia if you have been sick a short time and you are still able to cooperate with treatment in your own home. It may be that you are not sure you are ill or that you are unable to take your medicine regularly because you are forgetful. You can still be given Phase One treatment if you have someone in your family, or a friend who will remind you when you should take your medicine.

We suggest you take either nicotinic acid or nicotinamide* as your basic medicine, as both vitamins have the same effect on you. Both substances are B vitamins; nicotinamide was once called vitamin B-$_3$ Nicotinic acid (this is also called niacin) has an advantage which nicotinamide (also called niacinamide) does not have. It lowers the fatty substances, cholesterol and fatty acids in the blood. These substances play a role in hardening of the arteries. Since hardening of the arteries (arteriosclerosis) can lead to high blood pressure and

* In Canada and the U.S.A. 500 mgm. (half-gram) tablets are available. These are preferable to 100 mgm. tablets since it is simpler to take 6 tablets each day and the larger tablets contain less inert bulky fillers. In Great Britain patients will have to make special arrangements with their chemists to obtain them in the half-gram strength.

§189

senile changes in the brain, it may be desirable to use nicotinic acid in cases where these additional changes are present.

We have to start with one. If we start with nicotinic acid
you will be given a prescription for one month's supply at a
dose level of three grams per day. They are available in one-
half gram tablets. You will take two half-gram tablets after
each meal. The first time you take them you will probably
have a marked flush. About one-half to one hour after you
take the tablets you will become aware of a tingling sensation
in your forehead. Then your face will turn red and you will
feel hot and flushed. The flush will spread down your body.
Usually it will include your arms and chest, but very rarely
will your whole body flush. There is no need to be alarmed.
This is a normal reaction to this vitamin. There is no change
in your blood pressure and you will not faint.

You will be uncomfortable the first time and you might be
wise to take the first tablets in the evening while lying down
in bed. Each time you take the pills the reaction becomes less
strong and, within a few days to a few weeks, you will have
become accustomed to them. Eventually, as long as you take
the medicine regularly, you will stop flushing altogether, or
it will be so mild it will not trouble you. Some patients like
to take the nicotinic acid right after meals.

Sometimes patients are bothered by the acidity of nicotinic
acid. If this happens to you, you can take one-half a teaspoon
of bicarbonate of soda with the tablets. If, however, after you
have taken nicotinic acid regularly as prescribed, and you are
troubled by it, you may be advised to stop it and to take
nicotinamide instead. Nicotinamide produces no flush at all,
and for this reason it may be preferable for some patients. It
does not lower cholesterol, but can cause some nausea.

The treatment you would be on would, in addition, depend

on how old you are and what other physical complaints you may have.

For children thirteen years of age and younger, we prescribe one gram of nicotinamide for each fifty pounds of body weight. Children do not like the flush and it is difficult to persuade them to stay on nicotinic acid. They must stay on the vitamin until they are twenty-one years of age.

For patients aged fourteen to sixty-five, we prescribe either nicotinic acid or nicotinamide at the beginning. If either vitamin produces any unpleasant side effects, we prescribe the other. If you have a history of coronary disease, for example, or if there is a marked rise in blood cholesterol level, in your case we would prescribe nicotinic acid, for it lowers cholesterol, reduces high blood pressure and slows up the process of hardening of the arteries. Or if you have a history of peptic ulcer we would prefer nicotinamide, but nicotinic acid can also be used, for it can be obtained in a buffered form.

For all patients in this age group, we prescribe the vitamin for a year, and if the patient has a relapse, we prescribe it for another five years. We prefer nicotinic acid for everyone over age sixty-five because of its effect in lowering fat in blood.

You will continue on this treatment between one to three months. There is no point in taking smaller doses. If within this treatment period you show substantial improvement, then you will be advised to keep taking the medicine for one year, when it can be stopped on a trial basis. If you remain well you will not need to start again unless the symptoms you had originally begin to come back.

We teach patients in this group, as all patients, to be alert for signs of recurring illness. We might tell you, for example, if you have dizzy spells, as you did before, or if you find yourself becoming depressed once again, or notice any of the changes of perception which you experienced during your illness, to resume taking the full dose of vitamin without delay. For the sooner treatment begins, the better chance you have of remaining well. If such a relapse occurs you should stay on the vitamin for at least another five years. We have found that very few patients get sick again if they take their medicine regularly.

If you are very tense and anxious, we sometimes prescribe other medicines to help you over this stage.†

Both nicotinic acid and nicotinamide are compatible with any other treatment you may need if you should develop any other sickness. For example, if you should develop an infection, any treatment your doctor may recommend will not be interfered with by these vitamins. If you are pregnant you need not worry that the vitamins will harm your baby. Research with animals by our colleague, the late Professor M. Altschul, proved nicotinic acid did not injure rat infants. Recent work suggests that nicotinic acid given to pregnant women might have prevented their babies from being harmed by thalidomide.

But certain medicines are dangerous for schizophrenics and should not be taken. These are amphetamine, preludin and *some* antidepressants. We have seen schizophrenia return because patients were given amphetamine to help them lose weight.

We encourage our patients to put on weight if possible, and do not allow reducing diets at this stage of treatment, because of the danger of relapse. One of our patients who began putting on weight as she recovered was placed on Dexadrine by her family doctor when she became twenty

† Simple barbiturates, simple anti-anxiety compounds, such as meprobamate, diazepoxide, etc., or even the stronger tranquilizers, such as chlorpromazine or some of the other tranquilizers in common use today, may be prescribed.

pounds overweight. The gain in weight was a good sign but her doctor did not know that, nor did he know the danger of reducing pills for schizophrenics. As a result, her illness came back.

Of course, as a patient on our treatment program, you will have had a complete physical examination. If your teeth are infected, you will have had something done about it. Any source of chronic infection should be removed or treated. If there are hormone deficiencies, this will have been corrected.

If you are following this treatment, and if your disease has been caught early, in all likelihood you will get well without having to enter Phase Two. If you have not made a sufficient recovery in Phase One treatment, if you have been sick for too long, or if your schizophrenia is so severe it would throw too heavy a burden on you and your family to treat you at home, you will be required to come into hospital for Phase Two treatment.

PHASE TWO TREATMENT

In hospital you will continue to take one of these vitamins as before but, in addition, you will receive a short series of electroconvulsive therapy, ECT for short.

ECT is popularly called shock treatment, but this is the wrong name for it. The patient does not have his sensibilities shocked, feels no pain, and suffers no loss of blood or decrease in blood pressure. In this treatment small quantities of electricity are passed across the temples. As soon as the current is started the patient falls into a deep sleep and then has a convulsive seizure, but he is no more aware of it than he would be if he were having his tonsils out. He becomes aware of his surroundings some minutes later, but it may take several hours before he is fully awake and alert. This treatment is safe, painless and one of the most useful treatments developed in psychiatry.

The word "shock," since it is misleading and frightening, is better not used because it makes patients and families unnecessarily afraid. Some have preferred to call it electrotherapy, or ET, and this seems correct, but ECT is more specific.

You will have between six and twelve treatments of ECT at the rate of three treatments a week until the series is completed. There is no rule about it. The number will depend upon your rate of improvement. We ourselves give it without anaesthetics and muscle relaxants unless there is a special need for these.

After the last ECT is given, you will be watched carefully for seven to ten days. If you have shown improvement, and if it continues after this period is past, we feel optimistic that it will go on for as long as you take the vitamin. Nicotinic acid or nicotinamide should then be continued for one year as in Phase One treatment.

In some cases, if we feel that ECT should not or cannot be given, we prescribe tranquilizers instead, but we use half the usual dose, as the vitamin increases the sedative effect of the tranquilizers.

If you are cured with the combination of tranquilizers and vitamin, you will be discharged, and the tranquilizer dosage gradually reduced after several months. Our goal is to have you eventually get along on nicotinic acid or nicotinamide alone. There are very few patients who cannot do so after such treatment. If the symptoms come back at any time during this period, we will increase the tranquilizer dosage, and try again later to reduce it until it is no longer required.

Most patients recover after Phase Two treatment, but some do not, and they then enter Phase Three, when we add penicillamine, a breakdown product of penicillin, to the other treatment, together with a bit more ECT. In Phase Three about half the patients who failed Phase Two will recover.

PHASE THREE TREATMENT

This phase starts if you are not recovered, or not much improved, ten days after the last ECT has been given in Phase Two. We will then give you two grams of penicillamine a day for ten days, or until you develop a skin rash and a fever of 103 F. The fever may occur any time during the ten days and if it does, we will stop the penicillamine. Usually the temperature will be normal next day.

If this allergic reaction does not occur, we will continue treatment for the full period of ten days. You would, meanwhile, be taking your full daily dose of nicotinic acid, and given three to five more ECT treatments. If you recover, you will continue on the vitamin as in Phase One and Phase Two.

If, after this treatment has been completed, you do not improve, it is because you have been sick so long that the disease has become chronic, and treatment will have to continue for a long period of time, either in hospital or at home. As a rule, patients who have been sick for many years will not be helped with nicotinic acid alone. But if they can be improved in any way whatsoever, it is better to keep them on this treatment.

Finally, we will make every effort to get you well, for no matter how sick you are, or how long you have been sick, you have a chance for recovering and we will not deprive you of this chance.

*Appendix D*

GERIATRIC NUTRITION

Contrary to popular opinion, there is no difference between good nutrition for the elderly and for the mature adult. The vitamin and mineral requirements of the aged and the young are not materially different. Basic nutrition requirements for satisfactory metabolism do not change in a lifetime. However, there are many problems inherent in sound geriatric nutrition, which will be briefly discussed as follows:

1. As we grow older, we become "more set" in our eating habits. Dietary patterns of long standing are not changed easily. We must remember that each of us is the sum total of our past experiences, so prejudice, self-indulgence, taste preference, fear of certain foods and indifference all influence our selections of what we eat.

2. Obesity is a problem, since many oldsters diminish their physical activities and fewer calories are needed for energy. Underweight is no more desirable than obesity, so the regulation of the caloric intake to conform with normal body weight is important to sound geriatric nutrition.

3. Economic factors cause many older persons to eat the cheaper carbohydrate foods and omit the more expensive protein foods. Those who live alone frequently indulge in the cheaper packaged bakery goods which require no preparation and have little nutritional value.

4. Most old people do not have good teeth. Some of them, without teeth, have no dentures, or poorly fitted and uncomfortable ones, so foods cannot be properly masticated for digestion. This causes essential foods, such as meats and bulk fruits and vegetables, to be excluded from the diet.

5. Dietary habits and ill-health may cause the secretions in the gastrointestinal tract to decrease, making digestion and absorption more difficult. Constipation resulting from too

§199

little intake of fluids, fruits, and vegetables forming bulk, is a frequent complaint of the aged.

Physicians who have specialized in geriatric nutrition recommend that in later years the best diet is one high in proteins, moderate in carbohydrates, relatively low in fats, and *high in vitamins and minerals.*

Fluid intake—water, juices, milk, coffee and tea, when permitted—is generally too low and should be gradually increased daily. Many older individuals are on a salt-restricted diet because of cardiovascular troubles, and the loss of salt by perspiration or fever may present a critical condition for such persons.

When an elderly person refuses to drink milk, it may be easier to include dried skim milk in soup than to insist on milk drinking. Cheese dishes may supply the needed calcium and phosphorus. Ground meat and finely chopped vegetables are usually preferred by those with chewing difficulties.

Here are some recommended menus for the aged:

## SUGGESTED GERIATRIC MENU
### —INEXPENSIVE

*Breakfast*
>    Fruit or fruit juice
>    Cooked cereal with milk
>    Coffee or tea (when permitted)

*Lunch*
>    Soup with crackers
>    Egg or cheese sandwich
>    Vegetable
>    Beverage

*Dinner*
>    Hamburger steak
>    Salad, either fruit or vegetable

Two vegetables
Bread (one slice) and butter (one pat)
Beverage

*Bedtime Snack*
Milk or cheese with two or three crackers

## SUGGESTED GERIATRIC MENU
—MORE EXPENSIVE

*Breakfast*
Fruit juice or fruit
Two eggs and one piece of buttered toast
Milk

*Lunch*
Hot beef or ham sandwich
Pineapple and cottage cheese salad
Vegetable
Pudding
Beverage

*Dinner*
Fruit cocktail
Tender, small steak
Two vegetables
Roll and butter (one pat)
Cheese or ice cream (small serving of either)
Beverage

*Bedtime Snack*
Soft fruit or milk and two or three crackers

## SUGGESTED GERIATRIC MENU
—MORE EXPENSIVE

*Breakfast*
Sliced orange or sliced banana

Cooked cereal with milk
Soft-boiled egg with toast and butter (one pat)
Coffee or tea (if permitted)

*Lunch*

Soup with crackers
Cottage cheese salad—with pear or tomato
Vegetable
Ground-beef patty
Beverage

*Dinner*

Fruit salad
Two vegetables
Sliced chicken
Roll and butter (one pat)
Beverage

*Bedtime Snack*

Milk with two or three crackers, or small apple or pear

## SUGGESTED GERIATRIC MENU
—MORE EXPENSIVE

*Breakfast*

Fruit juice or half-grapefruit
Cooked cereal with milk
Toast (one piece), butter (one pat), and jelly
Coffee or tea (when permitted)

*Lunch*

Tomato and lettuce salad
Two soft-boiled eggs with toast or roll and butter (one pat)
Small serving of cheese
Vegetable
Beverage

*Dinner*
> Lean ground beef
> Two vegetables
> Applesauce
> Milk

*Bedtime Snack*
> Either a banana, dried cooked fruit, slice of pineapple,
> or half-cantaloupe

SUMMARY

We may summarize the requirements of good nutrition for geriatrics as follows:

1. *Lean meat, fish, or poultry*

Two servings daily. Sometimes, when finances allow only one serving of meat, fish, or poultry daily, peanut butter, cheese, or eggs may be substituted.

2. *Eggs*

A minimum of four or five eggs a week should be served.

3. *Vegetables*

Two helpings of vegetables daily, one of which should be a green, leafy, or dark-yellow vegetable.

4. *Fruits*

Two helpings a day. Citrus fruit, apples, pears, bananas, berries, cantaloupe, and other fruits are recommended.

5. *Milk*

Doctors say that adults should have a pint of milk daily. This requirement may be met by eating cheese, puddings, custards, soups, and other foods containing milk.

As we have seen, sound geriatric nutrition must be practiced if we are to retain our mental faculties as long as we live.